American College of Physicians

HOME CARE GUIDE
for
HIV and AIDS

FOR FAMILY AND FRIENDS GIVING CARE AT HOME

ALSO AVAILABLE FROM THE AMERICAN COLLEGE OF PHYSICIANS

American College of Physicians Home Care Guide for Cancer

Publications from the BMJ Publishing Group are available to members through the American College of Physicians.

Our *Resources for Internists* catalog and ordering information for the American College of Physicians and BMJ Publishing Group are available from:

Customer Service Center
American College of Physicians
Independence Mall West
Sixth Street at Race
Philadelphia, PA 19106-1572
215-351-2600
800-523-1546, ext. 2600

American College of Physicians

HOME CARE GUIDE
for
HIV and AIDS

FOR FAMILY AND FRIENDS GIVING CARE AT HOME

EDITOR
Peter S. Houts, PhD

ASSOCIATE EDITORS
Julia A. Bucher, RN, PhD
Francine P. Damianos, RN, MS
W. Christopher Ehmann, MD
Miriam Jacik, MSN
Elizabeth A. Johnston, RN, BSN
Margaret Kreher, MD
Arthur M. Nezu, PhD
Christine Maguth Nezu, PhD
John J. Zurlo, MD

CONTRIBUTORS
Carole A. Bean
Elise M. Givant, RN, OCN
Kathy B. Kambic, RN, OCN
Eric J. Pfeiffer, MS
Dale B. Schelzel, RN, OCN
Sandra J. Spoljaric, RN, OCN
Georgia L. Trostle, RN, BSN
Glenda M. Trumpower, MSW

HIV and AIDS PROJECT COORDINATOR
Marion M. Markowicz, MSS

A|C|P

Acquisitions Editor: Mary K. Ruff
Manager, Book Publishing: David Myers
Administrator, Book Publishing: Diane M. McCabe
Production Supervisor: Allan S. Kleinberg
Production Editor: Vicki Hoenigke
Interior and Cover Design: Colleen Woods-Esposito

Printed in the United States of America.
Composition by Fulcrum Data Services, Inc.
Printing/binding by Port City Press.

American College of Physicians
Independence Mall West
Sixth Street at Race
Philadelphia, PA 19106-1572

Library of Congress Cataloging in Publication Data

Home care guide for HIV and AIDS : how to care for family and friends at home / editor, Peter S. Houts; associate editors, Julia A. Bucher . . . [et al.]; contributors, Carole Bean . . . [et al.] ; HIV and AIDS project coordinator, Marion Markowicz.
    p.   cm.
  ISBN 0-943126-54-1 (alk. paper)
  1. AIDS (Disease)—Patients—Home care—Handbooks, manuals, etc.
I. Houts, Peter S.
  [DNLM: 1. HIV infections—nursing—handbooks. 2. HIV Infections—psychology—handbooks. 3. Home Nursing—methods—handbooks. WY 49 H7646 1998]
RC607.A26H655 1998
362.1'969792—DC21
DNLM/DLC
for Library of Congress   96–37121
                                           CIP

98 99 00 01 02 03 / 9 8 7 6 5 4 3 2 1

Acknowledgments

Many persons have contributed to the development of the *Home Care Guide for HIV and AIDS*—in particular, the HIV and AIDS patients and their families receiving care at the Milton S. Hershey Medical Center of the Pennsylvania State University College of Medicine. They have helped by telling us their problems and what was helpful in dealing with those problems, by reviewing what we wrote, and by showing us through their enthusiasm, fortitude, and courage that coping with HIV and AIDS can, with all of its difficulties, bring out the best in people and be an opportunity for growth.

The *Home Care Guide for HIV and AIDS* built on work done for an earlier book, the *Home Care Guide for Cancer.* The many people who are listed in its Acknowledgments section have indirectly contributed to this volume as well. We are indebted to them for the foundation of this work.

Three external reviewers have played an important part in refining this book. Anne Hughes, RN, MN, CS, OCN, Pamela Ryan, MSW, and Cynthia Leeder, RN, MS, CNS, gave extensive and detailed feedback on drafts and contributed substantially to the quality of this effort. Their help is very much appreciated. We also appreciate the editorial help of Daniel Cupper.

CONTENTS

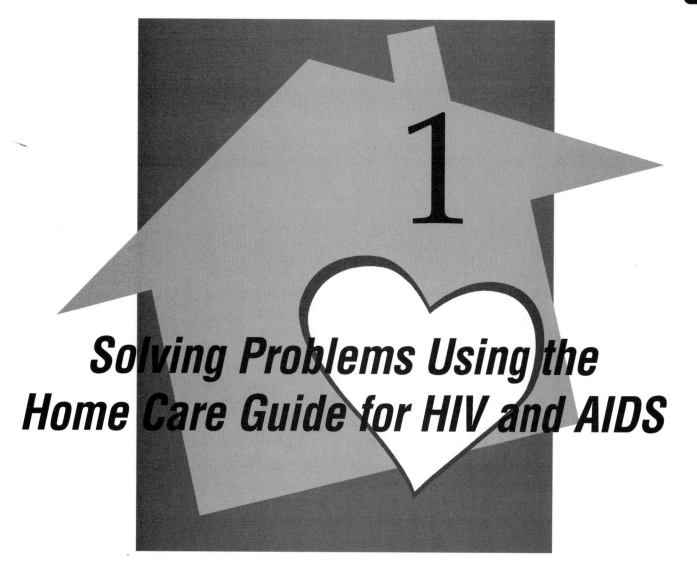

Solving Problems Using the Home Care Guide for HIV and AIDS

Solving Problems Using the Home Care Guide for HIV and AIDS

This book is for family, friends, and volunteers who are caring for persons with HIV/AIDS at home. It gives the information they need to solve caregiving problems while working cooperatively with a team of health professionals, such as nurses, physicians, and social workers, who are members of a hospital, outpatient, home health, or hospice team.

The book was written and edited by nurses, physicians, social workers, and psychologists who work in HIV/AIDS care, with help from family caregivers and volunteers.

HOW THE BOOK IS ORGANIZED

Each chapter is a *plan* on how to deal with problems that may occur when one is providing care at home. Each chapter covers five major topics:

1. *Understanding the Problem*: What the problem is, who is most likely to have it, when they might have it, what steps can be taken to help, and what is a realistic goal when dealing with the problem

2. *When To Get Professional Help*: When to call immediately, when to call during office hours, what information to have ready when you call, and what to say

3. *What You Can Do To Help*: How to deal with the problem and how to prevent the problem from occurring

4. *Possible Obstacles*: Misinformation and attitudes that can interfere with carrying out the plan and how to deal with it

5. *Carrying Out and Adjusting Your Plan*: How to check on whether you are making progress, how fast to expect change, and what to do if the plan isn't working

The chapters, called *home care plans,* in the *Home Care Guide for HIV and AIDS* deal with only the most common problems of persons with HIV/AIDS and their home caregivers. For other problems, you can use these chapters as models for the kinds of information you need to have for effective problem solving.

HOW TO MAKE THE BEST USE OF THE HOME CARE PLANS

Read key information headings first

The second page of each chapter is an overview, or a road map, of the contents of that chapter. In the chapter, topics are summarized in bold-face type, with information about the topic in regular type. An arrow appears in front of topics that are actions you can take or symptoms you should look for. By first reading the overview page, then the section "Understanding the Problem," and then just the boldface type (especially when there is an arrow in front of it), you can quickly and easily understand the problem and how you can deal with it. You can read the text, which is in regular-sized type, later when you need to understand the reasons for the recommendations in the chapter.

Read chapters before problems develop

By reading the chapters, or *plans,* before problems develop or become severe, home caregivers will be prepared when they do happen. Because some chapters include information on how to prevent problems, home caregivers may even prevent some problems from occurring. Also, most problems are easier to solve when they are just beginning, so early intervention can prevent problems from becoming serious.

Re-read chapters when problems persist

The chapters in the *Home Care Guide for HIV and AIDS* contain many ideas and strategies for dealing with caregiving problems, and it is hard to remember them all. Therefore, it is a good idea to re-read the chapters about problems that persist—to be sure that you are doing everything you can.

Use the home care plans as part of an orderly approach to problem solving

The *Home Care Guide for HIV and AIDS* by itself does not ensure effective problem solving. You need to develop your own plan to carry out the recommendations in this guide. The next section discusses how to solve problems using the home care plans.

Solving problems using the home care plans

Four key approaches that will help you to be effective in solving caregiving problems and to make the best use of the home care plans in this book:

1. Being **creative** in dealing with obstacles.

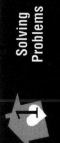

2. Being both **optimistic** and realistic in involving the ill person in the plan.

3. Developing an orderly **plan**.

4. Making effective use of **expert information**—the kind of information that is included in the *Home Care Guide for HIV and AIDS*.

You can remember these four key approaches by thinking of the word COPE (which means to succeed in solving problems):

C for Creativity

O for Optimism

P for Planning

E for Expert information

Research has shown that people who use the four COPE techniques are better problem solvers. Research has also shown that people who use the four COPE techniques experience less stress when dealing with problems.

These four approaches, in detail, are as follows:

Be CREATIVE

As a caregiver, you will be constantly challenged to think creatively. Each person is unique, and each problem is unique. Therefore, you must be creative in adapting your plans to fit each unique situation.

Most plans will run into obstacles or roadblocks. Overcoming these obstacles will also challenge your creativity. *When your plans do not work out as you had hoped, you should see this as a challenge to your creativity.*

Here are four ways of helping yourself think creatively when dealing with obstacles:

1. **See the obstacle from someone else's point of view**. Put yourself in the shoes of another person who can look at your problem differently and ask yourself what he or she would do.

2. **Ask for advice from others**. Ask other people who have faced similar problems for ideas on how to get around your obstacle.

3. **Determine how important or serious the obstacle really is**. Does this obstacle really interfere with your plan? Sometimes you can ignore or work around an obstacle and still carry out your plan.

4. **Brainstorm**. Think of as many ideas as you can. Do not worry if the ideas seem unrealistic, or even silly. Make the longest list that you can. Then review it to see if you can combine ideas into even better ideas. Finally, go over the list and select those ideas that will help the most and are feasible.

Have an OPTIMISTIC attitude while being realistic about your problems

Being optimistic means having a positive attitude and expecting to succeed. This is important for both the people with HIV/AIDS and their caregivers.

➤ Have a positive attitude.

One of the most important ways of helping the person you are caring for is to have a positive attitude. People who have HIV/AIDS need encouragement, and they need help noticing good experiences. The home care plan "Creating and Maintaining Positive Experiences" (Chapter 19) offers suggestions on how to provide this encouragement. At the same time, it is important to be realistic about the seriousness of the problems of the person you are caring for, so that he does not feel that his problems are being ignored or belittled.

➤ Expect to succeed.

If you think that there is a good chance of succeeding, you will do your best to carry out your plans. If you think the problem is hopeless and that nothing will work, it will be hard for you to do your best, and the people who are around you will also become discouraged. If you *do* feel discouraged and negative, then get help from someone who has a positive attitude and who is a good problem solver. This could be the person you are caring for, friends or family members, or health professionals. Read the home care plan "Coping with Depression" (Chapter 17) for help in controlling negative thinking, because negative thinking tends to interfere with effective problem solving.

➤ Take breaks from caregiving.

Do things that you enjoy to maintain a positive outlook, even when you feel under stress. Read the home care plan "Caregiving" (Chapter 2) for ideas and guidance about how to deal with your feelings as a caregiver. Also, the home care plans "Creating and Maintaining Positive Experiences" (Chapter 19), "Getting Companionship and Support" (Chapter 20), "Coping with Depression" (Chapter 17), and "Coping with Anxiety" (Chapter 18) apply as much to you as they do to the person with HIV/AIDS. Read and use those chapters for yourself. They will help you to have the emotional strength you need to keep a positive attitude and to solve the problems that come with caregiving.

Develop an orderly and systematic PLAN

Problem solving is done best in an orderly, systematic way. This means that you should do the following:

> ## Get the facts.

Be clear about what is happening. Separate facts from opinions.

> ## Review what you can do.

Read the home care plan and other written information about the problem. Ask health professionals for recommendations. Think back over your own experiences for ideas and strategies that worked in the past. Ask what you can reasonably hope to achieve.

> ## Decide on the best strategy.

Compare the advantages and disadvantages of the different approaches you could take, and develop a strategy that will give you a reasonable chance of achieving your goal.

> ## Consider obstacles.

Think of what could interfere with your plan, and think creatively about what you can do to deal with those obstacles.

> ## Carry out and adjust your plan.

Set deadlines for yourself to make sure things get done. Keep records of how the plan is working. This will help you to monitor progress and to explain to professional staff what you have done and what the results were. If the plan is not working or you are not having as much success as you had hoped, ask yourself if you are expecting change too fast and whether you should adjust your goals. Then repeat the problem-solving steps to develop a new plan, paying special attention to maintaining a positive attitude and expecting success.

Get EXPERT INFORMATION about the problem and what you can do about it

The foundation for good problem solving is knowledge about the problem and how to deal with it. *The* Home Care Guide for HIV and AIDS *contains the information you need to solve 22 common problems in home care.* To deal with problems other than those discussed in this book, you should try to obtain information on

1. *Understanding the Problem*: What the problem is, who is most likely to have it, and what can be done to help

2. *When To Get Professional Help*: When to call for help immediately, when to call during office hours, and what information to have ready when you call

3. *What You Can Do To Help*: How to deal with the problem and how to prevent it

---

4. *Possible Obstacles*: What can interfere with carrying out your plan

5. *Carrying Out and Adjusting Your Plan*: How to check on whether the plan is working and what to do if it is not

A note about spiritual problems

After being diagnosed with HIV/AIDS, and especially if death approaches, both the people who have this disease and their caregivers often ponder spiritual questions:

- Where did I come from?

- Why am I here?

- What is really important in my life?

- What happens after death?

These are questions that each person must answer within the framework of his or her beliefs, values, and experiences. Therefore, there is no chapter in this book on solving spiritual problems. However, a discussion on how to support someone who is pondering these very important issues is given in the chapter "Caregiving" (Chapter 2).

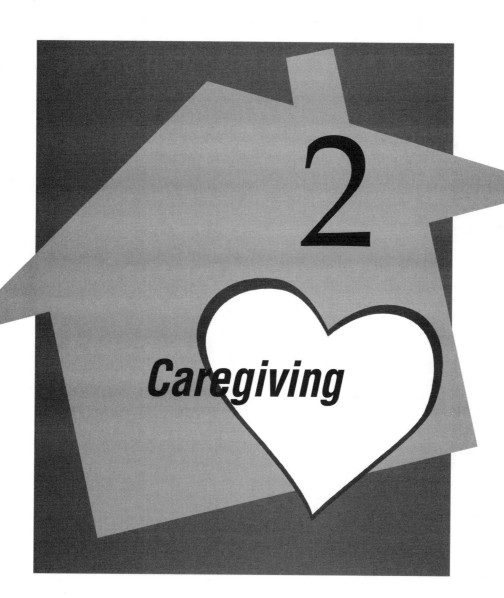

Caregiving

2

Caregiving

Overview of the Home Care Plan for *Caregiving*

 1. LEARNING HOW TO BE A CAREGIVER

   Caregivers work to solve problems

   Caregivers work as a member of a team

   Caregivers work to have a positive attitude toward caregiving

   Caregivers take care of themselves

   Your goals

 2. WHEN TO GET PROFESSIONAL HELP FOR YOURSELF

3. WHAT YOU CAN DO TO BE A SUPPORTIVE CAREGIVER

   Communicate effectively with the person you are caring for

   Give support for spiritual concerns

   Work with health care professionals

   Work with others who also care about the person

   Take care of your own needs and feelings

 4. POSSIBLE OBSTACLES

5. CARRYING OUT AND ADJUSTING YOUR PLAN

   Checking on results

   What to do if your plan does not work

Topics that have an arrow (➤) in front
of them are actions you can take or
symptoms you can look for.

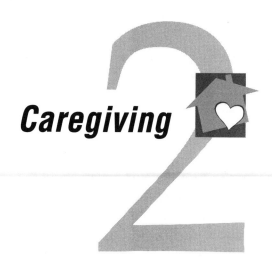

Caregiving

1. LEARNING HOW TO BE A CAREGIVER

Caregivers work to solve problems

Caregivers are problem solvers. You have been solving problems throughout your life. The only difference now is that many of the problems that come with HIV/AIDS are new to you and to the person you are helping. The *Home Care Guide for HIV and AIDS* will help both of you to solve these new problems; it will give you information and guidance organized into steps.

The plans are designed to help you solve problems, but you and the person with HIV/AIDS are the ones who will actually solve the problems. *You* decide what actions to take. *You* carry out the plans and adjust the plans to meet your special needs. *You* keep track of how well the plans are working and make changes as needed. Sometimes you will also need to develop new plans on your own to deal with problems that are not discussed in this book.

You and the person you are caring for are in charge of dealing with your problems. You are not people who are simply following instructions but are people who are making decisions and taking action.

Caregivers work as a member of a team

Good caregiving is not done alone—it requires a team of people with different skills and perspectives. Physicians, nurses, social workers, and clergy make important and unique contributions to care. But family members, friends, and volunteers are also important contributors. You have (or will develop) a close, personal relationship with the person who is ill—so you play a key role in involving the ill person in his or her care. Your close personal relationship helps you to understand and interpret the feelings, desires, and needs of the person who is ill. And, very importantly, you are the first to become aware of many physical and emotional problems and the first to deal with those problems; often you are the person who carries out the plans that you and other team members develop.

As a team member, your job is to work cooperatively with other members of the team in solving caregiving problems. To do this, you need to use the COPE problem-solving methods. You need to collect facts and develop an understanding about the disease, get expert information or guidance on actions to take, develop a plan about the disease, and then *carry out* that plan while keeping other members of the team informed. Most important, you need to have an optimistic and realistic attitude, and, as much as possible, you should keep the person you are caring for informed about and involved in his or her care.

Caregivers work to have a positive attitude toward caregiving

Emphasize the positive aspects of caregiving. For example, some successful caregivers see their work as helping someone they love and care deeply about. Others see caregiving spiritually ("I think this is part of God's plan for me.") Others feel that caregiving has enriched their lives. Some caregivers see it as a challenge and as an opportunity to do the best job they can. Still others see caregiving as a way of showing appreciation for the love and care that they have received themselves.

Caregiving can have important benefits to the caregiver. Caring for someone can give you a sense of satisfaction and confidence. Family members who provide care often feel closer to each other and to the person who is ill. You may discover an inner strength that you may not even have realized you had.

You may also find new, rewarding friendships with other caregivers who are going through similar experiences. These friendships may develop by talking to other people who have faced the same problems, by meeting people at a support group, by meeting people who have volunteered to help with caregiving, and by renewing relationships with family members and friends who have grown apart but who are drawn together because of the illness.

Caregivers take care of themselves

Helping someone with a serious illness such as HIV/AIDS is a big responsibility, especially as the illness progresses. The person you are caring for can become very dependent on you. Often, you will need help to carry out your job as a home caregiver. Learn what help is available to you in the community and ask health care workers and clergy how you can get additional help. The home care plan "Getting Help from Community and Volunteer Groups" (Chapter 21) provides suggestions on how to go about *getting* additional help. The *more you take care of your own need for rest, food, recreation, and relaxation, the better you will be able to help*. The home care plans "Creating and Maintaining Positive Experiences" (Chapter 19) and "Getting

Companionship and Support" (Chapter 20) apply as much to you as to the person you are helping. Use the ideas in those guides for yourself to be able to do your best as a caregiver.

YOUR GOALS

Know when to get professional help for yourself

Communicate effectively with the person you are caring for

Give support for spiritual concerns

Work with health care professionals

Work with others who also care about the person

Take care of your own needs and feelings

 WHEN TO GET PROFESSIONAL HELP FOR YOURSELF

Ask for help from health professionals or from a member of the clergy if any of the following are true:

➤ **You are experiencing severe anxiety or depression.**

See the home care plans "Coping with Depression" (Chapter 17, pp 196–198) and "Coping with Anxiety" (Chapter 18, p 215) for a list of symptoms that indicate professional help is needed.

➤ **Communication between you and the person you are caring for has broken down or has become painful or difficult.**

The stresses that come with HIV/AIDS—physical, psychological, financial, and emotional—can hamper your ability to communicate with the person you are caring for. If your anxiety and stress levels have increased to the point where you are not able to talk openly about important issues, you should get professional help from a health professional, hospice staff member, home health staff member, counselor, or social worker.

➤ **Your relationship with the person you are caring for is clouded by a history of abuse, addiction, or conflict.**

If you have suffered verbal, mental, physical, or sexual abuse at the hands of the person you are caring for, or if the person you are caring for has a history of alcohol or drug addiction that has affected the relationship in the past, then you are likely to have serious problems in caregiving. Such caregivers already have strong and deep-seated feelings, usually built up over many years. This situation calls for professional help from the start.

➤ **You are feeling overwhelmed by your responsibilities as caregiver, and do not know whom to call to find out how to get extra help at home.**

This is a common concern. The home care plan "Getting Help from Community Agencies and Volunteer Groups" (Chapter 21) deals specifically with this problem. Also, ask for help from the clinic nurses; from the social workers who work at the clinic, doctor's office, or hospice; or from the visiting nurses. They can help you to get the help you need.

➤ **You are considering moving the person to a nursing home or other setting.**

Social workers who are experienced in working with persons with HIV/AIDS can help you think through this issue. They understand the kind of care that is needed by persons with HIV/AIDS as well as what services different settings offer. Physicians and nurses, especially home health nurses, can also be of help.

➤ **You are feeling depressed or lonely.**

See the home care plan "Coping with Depression" (Chapter 17) and "Creating and Maintaining Positive Experiences" (Chapter 19). They give guidance on dealing with depression and on recognizing the signs that professional help is needed.

3. WHAT YOU CAN DO TO BE A SUPPORTIVE CAREGIVER

> **HERE ARE FIVE STEPS YOU CAN TAKE TO BE A SUPPORTIVE CAREGIVER:**
>
> Communicate effectively with the person you are caring for
>
> Give support for spiritual concerns
>
> Work with health care professionals
>
> Work with others who also care about the person
>
> Take care of your own needs and feelings

Communicate effectively with the person you are caring for

This is your most important responsibility as a caregiver, and it can also be the most challenging. The person you are caring for has to deal with the physical effects of the disease and the medicines as well as with the psychological and social challenges of living with HIV/AIDS. This may make it difficult for him or her to participate in the home care plans. *Nonetheless, your job is to involve the person you are caring for as much as possible in making decisions and carrying out the plans.* You should support his or her efforts to deal with the reality of the prognosis emotionally. You can do this by

➤ **Helping the person you are caring for to accept that he or she has HIV/AIDS**

Some people with HIV/AIDS try to deal with upsetting news by pretending that it has not happened. This is known as "denial." Denial can be a normal response and healthy when it helps the person live as normal a life as possible. It *can* be harmful, however, if it leads him or her to do things that make the illness worse, such as avoiding taking medicines or engaging in activities that are physically harmful (for example, drug abuse).

Sometimes what looks like "denial" is actually the person's attempt to protect loved ones from the hard realities of the illness. If this is the case, you should reassure him or her that you are willing to listen and talk about all aspects of the illness—even though it may be hard for both of you.

Support the efforts of the person you are caring for to have as normal a lifestyle as possible. However, a "normal" lifestyle should *not* include engaging in potentially harmful activities. If he or she is pretending that "nothing is wrong," *you* need to remain clear-sighted—to help ensure that he or she is not taking health risks.

➤ **Creating a climate that encourages the sharing of feelings and that supports the ill person's efforts to share**

Talk about important or sensitive topics at a time and place that are calm and conducive to open communication—not in the midst of a crisis or a family argument. Think about when you have had important talks in the past and try to recreate that setting.

Communicate your availability. One of the most important messages you can communicate to the person with HIV/AIDS is "If you want to discuss this uncomfortable issue, I'm willing to do it." But leave the timing up to him or her. To the greatest extent possible, let decisions on what feelings to share and on when, how, and with whom to share them be made by the person you are caring for. At this time in the person's life, many issues and decisions are beyond his or her control. By not pressing the issue, you allow the person to retain control over this part of his or her life.

Caregiving 2

➤ Understanding that conflicts can arise when home caregivers are not family members

Sometimes families are estranged from the person with HIV/AIDS. They have not been in touch or are not talking. When the person with HIV/AIDS selects a home caregiver who is not a family member, conflicts can arise between this caregiver and the family. Any conflicts that arise between family members and others who want to be home caregivers should be resolved by asking the ill person what he or she wants and working out a compromise to that end. It is important to stress that a home caregiver need not be a family member. Whatever the relationship, the only requirement for being a caregiver are (1) an honest commitment to the ill person and (2) his or her desire and permission for you to help.

➤ Being realistic and flexible about what you hope to communicate or agree on

People with HIV/AIDS want to share many things, but they may not share all of them with the same person. Let the person you are caring for talk about whatever he or she wants with whomever he or she wants. It is OK if the person is not telling you everything, as long as he or she is telling somebody. Also, remember that he or she may have spent a lifetime developing a communication style and that this will not change overnight. Some people have never felt comfortable talking about their feelings. Try to accept that this will not change now.

Sharing does not always mean talking. The person with HIV/AIDS may feel more comfortable writing about his or her feelings or expressing them through an activity. He or she may express feelings in other nonverbal ways, such as by making gestures or facial expressions, touching, or just asking that you be present.

Remember that you do not have to agree. No two people are always going to see eye-to-eye. Although you and the person you are caring for may disagree on issues such as when, how, and what to share, remember that this is one of the patterns of life that cannot always be resolved.

➤ Helping the person you are caring for to deal with anxiety and depression

People with HIV/AIDS may become anxious about medical procedures, about the disease, or about the future. Their anxiety may also be a side effect of medicines they are taking or of the disease itself. The home care plan "Coping with Anxiety" (Chapter 18) can help the person you are caring for decide how to deal with such feelings.

Many people with HIV/AIDS also feel depressed at some time during the illness. The home care plan "Coping with Depression" (Chapter 17) gives advice on how to control depression, especially in its early stages. Both you and the person you are caring for should read these chapters and work together as a team.

When you and the person with HIV/AIDS disagree on important issues:

➤ **Explain your needs openly.**

Sometimes you may need to ask the person with HIV/AIDS to do something to make your life easier or make your caregiving responsibilities more manageable. Understand that conflict resolution does not always mean everyone is happy. On some issues you will have to give in; on others, the other person will need to give in.

➤ **Suggest a trial run or time limit.**

If you want the person you are caring for to try something new (such as a new bed or a certain medication schedule) and he or she is resisting, ask him or her to try it for a limited time—for example, for 1 week—and then to evaluate the situation. This avoids making the person feel locked into a decision. If, for example, the person resists writing a will or power of attorney, ask if he or she will at least read one over and discuss it.

➤ **Choose your battles carefully.**

Ask yourself: "What's really important here? Am I being stubborn on an issue because I need to win an argument or be in control?" Decide to try to avoid or ignore the minor conflicts and instead use your energy and influence for important issues.

➤ **Let the person you are caring for make as many decisions as possible.**

If the person you are caring for understands the consequences of a given decision, the caregiver should accept the person's right to make that decision. Taking away a person's ability to make decisions can undermine feelings of control, which interferes with the ability to deal with other aspects of this stressful illness.

Give support for spiritual concerns

Spiritual questions usually become important after physical, emotional, and social problems have been resolved or are under control. Therefore, by attending to nonspiritual problems, you are enabling the person you are caring for to begin to consider fundamental spiritual issues.

Spiritual concerns raise fundamental questions about life such as "Why are we here?" "What is a good life?" or "What happens after death?" These profound questions become especially important when dealing with a potentially terminal illness. As a caregiver, your job is to support the person you are caring for in thinking through his or her personal answers to these questions.

He or she may want to make sense of life experiences—to reminisce—to talk about the past and to look for meaning in what has happened. *As a caregiver, listening is the most important thing you can do to help.* You may also share your experiences and feelings, but your main way of helping is to listen!

Spiritual questions are not answered easily, and for many, definite answers are not possible. For those whose faith gives answers and solace, your support of that faith will be helpful and appreciated. For those who are troubled by uncertainty, you may help by sharing your own questions and uncertainties—thereby showing that their concerns are normal and reasonable.

Work with health care professionals

Below are some practical suggestions to keep in mind when you need information and help from health professionals.

> ➤ **Be clear about what you want and get to the point as soon as possible.**

Make lists of questions and concerns and have them in front of you when you are talking to health professionals. Have paper and pencil ready to make notes.

> ➤ **Have ready all the information health professionals may need when you call.**

Many of the home care plans have lists of information you should have ready when you call for professional help. For example, if the person you are caring for has a fever, have information ready on how much liquid was taken in over the past 8 hours and if any medicines were given to reduce the fever, and so on (see the home care plan "Fever and Infections" [Chapter 5]). Refer to the section "When you call, have the answers ready to the following questions" that appears in each chapter of this book for a specific list of information medical staff may need.

> ➤ **Bring lists of medicines to appointments.**

Make a list of the names of all medicines (including over-the-counter, nonprescription medicines) that the person you are caring for is currently taking and the times that they are given. Show this list to the health care professionals each time you meet for an appointment. Some drugs do not work well together and should not be given at the same time of day or perhaps should not be taken together at all. Health care professionals will check this list and advise you and the person you are caring for on what medication is best to take and at what times it should be taken.

➤ **Be firm and straightforward about getting the information and help you need.**

Professionals are there to help you to be a good caregiver. Make your requests with confidence that you will get the help you need. Feel free to say when you do not understand. Remain calm. Being angry is not usually helpful. Being pleasant, firm, and persistent and showing appreciation are usually the best strategies.

The home care plan "Getting Treatment Information" (Chapter 22) offers many good ideas about how to work effectively with medical staff. Read that plan and use those ideas.

Work with others who also care about the person

➤ **Do not try to do everything yourself. Ask for help.**

Family members, friends, clergy, and people who belong to community organizations can all help out. Some can help with planning, and others will just want to help in carrying out the plans and giving support.

Those who live in the same household or who are going to be very involved in carrying out the plans should participate in actually *creating* the plans and should read and understand the home care plans in this book. They will then be able to work with you and with the person you are caring for as part of a team. Also, if they have had a hand in the planning, they will be more committed to carrying out the plans.

Some people want to help, but they need to be told how. It is important to be clear with them about what you would like them to do and about the limits of what is expected of them.

The home care plan "Getting Help from Community Agencies and Volunteer Groups" (Chapter 21) provides suggestions on how community organizations and volunteers can help with many caregiving responsibilities.

Take care of your own needs and feelings

You need to be at your best if you are to do the best job of helping. *Therefore, you should pay attention to your own needs as well as those of the person you are helping.* Set limits on what you can reasonably expect yourself to do. You should take time off to care for yourself and your needs. And you should ask for help before stress builds up.

It is natural to have strong feelings when helping someone with a serious illness. The following is a list of common feelings that caregivers may have, and the strategies for dealing with these feelings if they become severe.

Feeling overwhelmed

Caregivers as well as the person with HIV/AIDS may feel overwhelmed and confused when they learn that the disease is progressing.

Here is how you can deal with feeling overwhelmed:

➤ **Try not to make important decisions while you are upset.**

Sometimes you must make decisions immediately, but often you do not need to. Ask the doctor, nurse, or social worker how much time you should take before making a particular decision.

➤ **Take time to sort things out.**

It is important to take some time to let your thinking become clear again. Different people need different amounts of time. Give yourself enough time to become more emotionally stable so that you can make plans and decisions with a clear mind and a more peaceful spirit.

➤ **Talk over important problems with others who are feeling more level-headed and rational.**

If you are feeling very upset or discouraged, ask a friend, neighbor, or family member to help. They can bring a calmer perspective to the situation as well as new ideas and help in dealing with the problems you are facing.

Anger

There will be many reasons for you to become angry while you are caring for a person with HIV/AIDS. For example, the person you are caring for may be demanding or irritating at times. Friends, family members, or professionals may not be as helpful or understanding as you would like them to be. Some people feel angry because their God seems to have somehow let them down. Others are angry at the disease itself. It is natural to be angry when your life feels like it has been turned upside down by a serious illness like HIV/AIDS.

These feelings are normal! It is all right to feel this way at times. It is what you *do* with your feelings that is important. The best way to deal with angry feelings is to recognize them, accept them, and find some way to express them appropriately. If you don't deal with your anger, it can get in the way of almost everything you do.

Here are ways you can deal with your anger:

➤ **Try to see the situation from the other person's point of view.**

Recognize that other people, including the person with HIV/AIDS, are under stress, too. People react in different ways to the stressful events in their lives. Some act out their fear, anger, or stress by striking out at others, especially those who are close to them.

➤ **Express your anger in an appropriate way before you feel it is out of control.**

If you wait, your anger may lead to actions and words that you may later regret. Anger that is out of control can cloud a person's good judgment.

➤ **Find safe ways to express your anger.**

This can include such things as beating on a pillow, hollering out loud in a car or in a closed room, or doing some hard exercise. Sometimes it helps to ventilate anger with someone who is "safe"—who will not be offended or strike back. Get away from the situation for a while and try to calm down before you go back and deal with what made you angry.

➤ **Try not to feel guilty about your anger.**

Anger is a natural response to a difficult situation. Guilt can make you feel that you are the only cause of the problem when in reality there are many causes. Guilt can get in the way of dealing with the real problem and with the ways that you express your anger.

➤ **Talk to someone about why you feel angry.**

Explaining to another person why you feel angry helps you to understand the reasons for your anger and why you reacted as you did.

Fear

You may become afraid when someone you care for deeply has a serious illness. You do not know what is in store for him or her or for yourself, and you may be fearful that you will not be able to handle what happens.

Here are ways you can deal with your fears:

> **Learn as much as possible about what is happening and what may happen in the future.**

This can reduce fear of the unknown and help you to be realistic so that you can prepare for the future. Talk with health professionals and with other people who have cared for someone with HIV/AIDS to see if you are exaggerating the problems and risks.

> **Talk to someone about your fears.**

It often helps to explain to an understanding person why you feel fearful. This helps you to think through the reasons for your feelings. Also, talking to an understanding person will show you that other people understand and appreciate how you feel.

> **Read the home care plan "Coping with Anxiety" (Chapter 18).**

The ideas and techniques in that chapter can be used by you *and* by the person with HIV/AIDS.

Loss and sorrow

A serious, life-threatening illness can bring on a great sense of loss and sorrow. You may feel sad that plans that you had for the future may not be fulfilled. You may feel the loss of the "normal" person and the "normal" things you did before this illness. Memories of how he or she used to be may make you sad. You may also feel burdened by more responsibilities that you have to deal with alone.

Here are ways you can deal with loss and sorrow:

> **Talk about your feelings of loss with other people who have had similar experiences.**

People who have been caregivers for persons with serious illnesses will usually understand how you feel. Support groups are one way to find people who have had similar experiences and who can understand and appreciate your feelings.

> **Read the home care plan "Coping with Depression" (Chapter 17).**

Feelings of loss are often part of feeling depressed. The ideas and techniques in this plan can be used by you as well as by the person you are caring for to help manage or prevent depression.

Guilt

Many people caring for someone with HIV/AIDS feel guilty at some time during the illness. They may feel guilty because they blame the person for his or her illness. They may feel guilty because they are well and the person whom they care about so deeply is sick. They may feel guilty for having caused or added to the problem. Or, they may feel guilty for not doing a better job of caring for and supporting the person with HIV/AIDS. They may feel guilty because they feel angry or upset with him or her. Some people feel guilt almost out of habit. They have learned from childhood to feel guilty when something goes wrong.

Although feeling guilty is understandable, it can interfere with doing the best possible job of caregiving. Guilt makes you think only about what *you* did wrong, while most problems have many causes and what you did is only part of the reason for the problem. To solve a problem, you have to look objectively at *all* of the causes and then develop plans to deal with the whole problem. For example, if you feel anger toward the person you are caring for, often this is partly because of what he or she did as well as what you did. To deal with the cause of the anger, you need to talk openly with him or her about what you both did. Feeling guilty will not the solve the problem.

Your goal here is to work toward forgiveness for yourself and for the other person. Dwelling on guilt feelings about the past will rob you of precious energy that you need to cope with the present.

Here are ways of dealing with guilt:

➤ **Talk to other people who have gone through similar experiences.**

It is often easier to see a situation objectively when it happens to someone else. This can give you perspective on your own problems.

➤ **Do not expect yourself to be perfect.**

Expecting perfection from yourself can cause guilt to be a regular part of your life. It is helpful to remember that you are human and that you will make mistakes from time to time.

➤ **Do not dwell on your mistakes.**

Accept your mistakes and get beyond them as best you can. The home care plan "Coping with Depression" (Chapter 17) offers useful ideas for controlling negative thoughts by replacing them with positive, creative thoughts.

Remember, you will be most effective in helping the person with HIV/AIDS when you feel your best. If feeling guilty makes you upset, it will interfere with your role as a caregiver by making you doubt yourself.

4. POSSIBLE OBSTACLES

Here are some attitudes, fears, and misconceptions that could prevent you from carrying out your plan

"The person I am caring for doesn't want to talk about his feelings."

Response: He is the best judge of that. Your job is to make sure that you are available to listen when and if he decides to talk about feelings.

"What if the person I am caring for talks about things that I don't want to hear?"

Response: Even if what you hear hurts you, consider it in the larger context of what it means to her to be able to express herself. Remember that you don't have to resolve everything. You are being helpful just by listening.

"The person I am caring for won't follow my advice."

Response: If you are feeling frustrated because the person you are caring for will not follow your advice, try to understand how important it is for him or her to retain some control. You may know what is best for the person you are caring for, but realize that your job is to be supportive, *not* to make decisions for him. If you have a dominant personality or have been the one to make decisions in your family, be prepared to practice letting go of control.

"I'm swamped with so many problems that I don't have time to take care of my *own* needs."

Response: This is the most common reason that caregivers become exhausted: They become so preoccupied with problems that they do not pay attention to themselves. *You will be a better caregiver in the long run if you take the time, especially when stress is high, to get help so that you can do things that you enjoy and that relax you.*

"If I don't do it, it won't get done."

Response: Learn to ask others for help. *You should also sort out things that really need to be done versus what you would like to see done.* It is OK to let some things, like housework, slide a bit when you take on new responsibilities.

"I hate to ask other people to help me."

Response: There are two ways of getting around this problem. You can get together socially with people who could help and let them volunteer or you could have someone else ask for help for you. *Read the home care plan "Getting Companionship and Support" (Chapter 20) for ideas about how to make visits from others pleasant and rewarding.* Then they will want to visit and help.

"The person I'm helping doesn't want other people to help us."

Response: Suggest trying to get help for just a short time, and then you both can talk over how it worked out. Also, *explain that you need help too.*

Think of other obstacles

Identify additional roadblocks that could keep you from following the recommendations of this home care plan.

- Will the person I am caring for cooperate?

- Will other people help?

- How can I explain my needs to other people?

- Do I have the time and energy to carry out my plan?

You need to develop plans for getting around roadblocks. Use the four COPE ideas (Creativity, Optimism, Planning, and Expert information) in developing your plans. See pp 4–8 for a discussion on how to use the four COPE ideas in overcoming your obstacles.

5. CARRYING OUT AND ADJUSTING YOUR PLAN

Carrying out your plan

Start using the ideas in the *Home Care Guide for HIV and AIDS* now. Do not wait until you feel overwhelmed. It is easier to develop good caregiving habits and attitudes early, before problems get out of hand.

It is especially important to begin work early on the home care plans "Creating and Maintaining Positive Experiences" (Chapter 19) and "Getting Companionship and Support" (Chapter 20). They apply to you, the caregiver, as much as they do to the person you are caring for. These chapters can give you the strength and resources to deal with stressful situations. Use them early so that you will have strength and support available when you need it.

Be realistic about what you expect of yourself. Do not expect to be perfect. Everyone makes mistakes. It takes time to learn to be a caregiver for someone with HIV/AIDS.

Ask others for help if there are some parts of caregiving that are especially difficult for you.

Be realistic in your expectations for sharing feelings. Most people do not change their styles of communicating quickly.

Checking on results

Every week or so you should take time to think about how you are doing as a caregiver. Look through this chapter and ask yourself how closely you are matching the "successful caregiver" that is described at the beginning of this plan.

What to do if your plan does not work

If you cannot do the things that are essential for the person you are helping, talk to a doctor, nurse, or social worker about getting the help that you need.

If you become so upset that your emotions interfere with your ability to perform your caregiving tasks, or if you are having severe depression or anxiety symptoms (see the home care plans "Coping with Depression" [Chapter 17] and "Coping with Anxiety" [Chapter 18]), then talk to the doctor, nurse, or social worker about getting help for yourself.

3

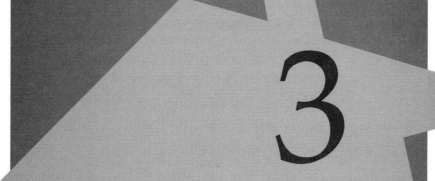

Preventing the Spread of HIV and Other Infections

Overview of the Home Care Plan for
Preventing the Spread of HIV and Other Infections

1. UNDERSTANDING THE PROBLEM

Fears about the transmission or spread of HIV

The known routes for the spread of HIV/AIDS

Your goals

2. WHEN TO GET PROFESSIONAL HELP FOR YOURSELF

Medical emergencies

Symptoms that do not indicate an emergency but should be reported

Information to have ready when you call

What to say when you call

3. WHAT YOU CAN DO TO HELP

Prevent getting HIV yourself

Keep the home environment clean and safe

Deal with your fears of becoming infected

Prevent the spread of other infections *to* the person with HIV/AIDS

4. POSSIBLE OBSTACLES

5. CARRYING OUT AND ADJUSTING YOUR PLAN

Checking on results

What to do if your plan does not work

Topics that have an arrow (➤) in front of them are actions you can take or symptoms you can look for.

Preventing the Spread of HIV and Other Infections

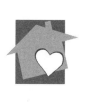

 UNDERSTANDING THE PROBLEM

Many people are concerned about the ways that HIV, the virus that causes AIDS, is spread. Caregivers need good information about the risk of acquiring HIV while helping someone who is HIV-positive or who has the disease AIDS.

Fears about the spread of HIV are usually greater than the actual degree of risk. HIV is spread through any of the following three known routes:

1. Contaminated blood and blood products

2. Sexual activity with a person who is HIV-positive

3. From an HIV-positive mother to her unborn or newborn child

The first route refers to receiving contaminated blood through a transfusion or from sharing contaminated needles that are used to inject medications such as steroids and insulin or to inject illicit drugs. There is *no* evidence that the AIDS virus is spread by insect bites, air, water, food, or close nonsexual contacts with a person who is HIV-positive. Caregivers of persons with HIV/AIDS are *not* at significant risk for becoming HIV-infected while caring for such indi-

> ➤ The information in this home care plan fits most situations, but yours may be different.
>
> ➤ If the doctor or nurse tells you to do something else, follow what he or she says.
>
> ➤ If you think there may be a medical emergency, see the section "When To Get Professional Help for Yourself" on pp 30–31.

viduals, provided that they take the proper precautions, which are described in this chapter.

The Centers for Disease Control and Prevention has developed guidelines to prevent the spread of HIV infection. These guidelines are the basis of the recommendations in this chapter.

Another concern is spreading other infections *to* persons with HIV/AIDS. This will also be discussed in this chapter.

YOUR GOALS

Know when to get professional help

Take care of yourself

Keep the home environment clean and safe

Deal with your fears of becoming infected

Prevent the spread of other infections to the person with HIV/AIDS

WHEN TO GET PROFESSIONAL HELP FOR YOURSELF

Caregivers who develop symptoms similar to those of HIV/AIDS may wonder whether they have contracted the virus. Sometimes they are concerned because they have engaged in activities (such as needle sharing or unprotected sexual contact) that have put them at risk. Signs and symptoms of HIV/AIDS can be similar to those of other illnesses. Consulting a doctor or nurse can clear up any doubts.

Medical emergencies

Call a physician immediately if you have been accidentally stuck with a contaminated needle or other sharp object, or if contaminated material comes in contact with an open cut or damaged skin. The physician may prescribe a medication, such as AZT (zidovudine), which may reduce the risk of becoming infected with HIV.

Symptoms that do not indicate an emergency but should be reported

Call the doctor or nurse if you have had any of the following symptoms for a month or longer:

➤ Temperatures of 99° to 101 °F not related to a cold or known infection

➤ Unusual fatigue not caused by overwork, insomnia, depression, or stress

➤ Weight loss not linked to dieting or an effort to lose weight

➤ Bouts of unexplained diarrhea

➤ Rash (cause unknown)

➤ Profuse night sweats

➤ Painless lumps in the groin, neck area, or armpits

➤ Ulcers or soreness in the mouth or throat that make eating painful

➤ Persistent vaginal "yeast" infections with white curdlike discharge and much itching.

➤ White plaques on the roof of the mouth

If the doctor, nurse, or you are concerned that you may be HIV-infected, a simple blood test can be performed. However, unless you have engaged in behavior that has put you at risk, the chance that you will become HIV-infected while caring for someone with HIV/AIDS is *extremely small*.

When you call, have the answers ready to the following questions:

1. At what time(s) each day does your temperature tend to rise? What is your temperature at these times?

2. Does fatigue prevent you from working or from other everyday activities? Do you sleep well?

3. Have you lost weight? If so, how much?

4. If you have diarrhea, what are the amount, frequency, color, and consistency of the stools?

5. If you have a rash, where is it located? What does it look like, and how does it feel?

6. Do you have night sweats every night? If so, how excessive is the sweating? (For example, do you have to change bed clothes during the night?)

7. If you have swollen lymph lands, where are they located? How many are there? Are they painful?

8. How does the throat, tongue, and inner portion of the mouth look? How painful is swallowing?

9. If you have a yeast infection, have you tried any over-the-counter medications?

Here is an example of what you might say when calling for professional help:

"I am John Davis, Adam Smith's caregiver. Adam is a patient of Dr. Black. Adam tested positive for HIV 6 months ago. Now *I'm* not feeling well. Each evening my temperature is 100 °F. I believe my fever breaks during the night because I sweat a great deal while I sleep and wake up exhausted each morning. I believe I may become HIV-infected myself, and would like to schedule an appointment for HIV testing."

3. WHAT YOU CAN DO TO HELP

> **HERE ARE FOUR STEPS YOU CAN TAKE TO MAKE CAREGIVING EASIER AND SAFER BOTH FOR YOURSELF AND FOR THE PERSON YOU ARE CARING FOR:**
>
> Prevent getting HIV yourself
>
> Keep the home environment clean and safe
>
> Deal with your fears of becoming infected
>
> Prevent the spread of other infections *to* the person with HIV/AIDS

Prevent getting HIV yourself

➤ **Use a proper container to dispose of sharp objects used by the person with HIV/AIDS.**

Place used needles, razors, and other sharp objects that may be contaminated with the AIDS virus into a rigid, nonbreakable, puncture-proof container. A coffee can with a lid or a sturdy detergent bottle will do. When the container is full, place a solution of one part bleach and 10 parts water into it to decontaminate the contents. Keep the lid on and tape it closed. Place the full container in the garbage can on the day of pickup. **Be sure to keep the container out of reach of children and away from other adults.**

➤ **Dispose of contaminated dressings properly.**

Dressings that have blood-stained drainage on them are contaminated. Place them in a sturdy plastic bag immediately and then into a second plastic bag before disposing of them in the garbage.

➤ **Wash your hands with soap and warm water after coming into contact with the body fluids of the person with HIV/AIDS.**

Hand washing is the most important means of preventing the spread of infection to yourself. Proper hand washing includes the use of warm water, plenty of soap, rubbing over all surfaces of both hands, and thorough rinsing. Wash hands immediately after being in contact with the body fluids of the person with HIV/AIDS, especially if these fluids contain the blood of the person with HIV/AIDS.

➤ **Wear disposable latex gloves when caring for the patient if you foresee that you will come in contact with blood or body fluids.**

Body fluids *known* to transmit HIV infection are blood, semen, vaginal secretions, and breast milk.

➤ **Wear rubber gloves when cleaning the bathroom.**

Rubber gloves protect your skin from coming into contact with any HIV-infected body fluids. Rinse the outside of the gloves after you remove them.

Special note for protecting babies of mothers with HIV/AIDS.

HIV-positive mothers of newborn infants should not breastfeed their children because the virus can be transmitted through breast milk.

➤ **Keep yourself in good health.**

Caring for someone with HIV/AIDS can be physically and psychologically taxing.

Caring for yourself is therefore very important. To provide the best care, you need to be healthy and alert. Make sure you get enough rest, eat healthy foods, exercise, and have time away from the person you are caring for. Take time for relaxation and fun so that you do not "burn out."

Keep the home environment clean and safe

A clean, safe home environment will protect both family members and the person with HIV/AIDS from contracting infections.

➤ **Keep the home well ventilated.**

Open the windows to allow fresh air into the home. A stuffy, damp home invites the growth of mold and fungus. These may be a source of infection to the person with HIV/AIDS. Fresh air and room deodorizers may also eliminate the smell of urine, vomit, and diarrhea.

> **Wash all laundry with detergent in hot or warm water.**

Washing clothes in this manner will destroy viruses. Clothes of the person with HIV/AIDS do not necessarily have to be washed separately. If linens and personal clothes are soiled with blood or other body fluids, add bleach to the soapy water.

> **Keep toothbrushes, towels, and razors of the person you are caring for separate from those of family members.**

The person with HIV/AIDS should have his or her own towel, washcloth, razor, and toothbrush to protect himself or herself from infections and also to protect family members from coming into contact with the HIV/AIDS virus. If there are others in the household who are HIV-positive, they should also have their own towels, washcloths, razors, and toothbrushes.

> **Wash dishes in hot, soapy water to protect everyone from infections.**

The person with HIV/AIDS does not need special dishes or utensils, nor do these need to be disposable. Routine washing of all dishes in the household with hot, soapy water will destroy viruses. Family members should not eat with the same unwashed utensils or drink from the same unwashed glass as the person with HIV/AIDS because they can easily transfer germs to the person with HIV/AIDS.

> **Clean up spills quickly and properly, especially if they include bloody drainage or other potentially infectious body fluids.**

Gloves can be worn when cleaning up spills of potentially infectious body fluids, especially when the spills cover large areas. Use paper towels to absorb the spill, and put them into a double plastic bag immediately. Wipe the area with a solution of 1 part bleach and 10 parts water. Have a container of this solution prepared and readily available for use. It is also wise to wipe down surfaces in the kitchen, bathroom, and bedroom often with the diluted bleach solution or disinfectant cleaners such as Lysol.

> **Keep the garbage can covered, and empty it often if contaminated materials have been placed in it.**

Keep a plastic lining or bag in the garbage can. Keep the lid on to keep mice, ants, flies, and roaches from attacking its contents. Empty the household garbage can whenever it is full and place contaminated contents in the outside garbage immediately.

➤ Dispose of sanitary napkins and tampons (of the person with HIV/AIDS) in containers with tight lids or double-bag them with plastic bags.

Deal with your fears of becoming infected

As the caregiver of a person with HIV/AIDS, you may worry that you have become infected with the virus. Such fears are usually unfounded unless:

➤ You have had sexual relations with a person who has HIV/AIDS and did not use a condom

➤ You have received a transfusion of a blood product that was untested and perhaps contaminated

➤ You have injected yourself with drugs using a contaminated syringe or needle

➤ You have had blood, bloody drainage, or saliva from the person with HIV/AIDS enter a cut or open area on your skin, mouth, or other body part

➤ You have been injured by a sharp object like a razor or needle used by the person with HIV/AIDS

The last two items are rarely the reason for acquiring HIV.

If any of the conditions listed above occur, you may want to be tested for HIV. The results of this blood test may ease your mind. Often persons who have been exposed to the AIDS virus, in one way or another, may need to be tested again in 3 months. Having two negative test results over a 6-month period usually means that you have not been infected with HIV. If you are still worried that you may have contracted the virus, talk to the doctor or nurse about your concerns. about becoming infected with HIV/AIDS.

Prevent the spread of other infections *to* the person with HIV/AIDS

The person with HIV/AIDS has poor ability to fight off new infections because of his or her failing immune system. You, the caregiver, can help reduce the risk of exposing the person with HIV/AIDS to new infections.

➤ If you have a cold, try to arrange for someone else to provide care.

Persons with HIV/AIDS are very susceptible to respiratory infections. If at all possible, try to arrange for someone else to provide care when you have a cold or other infection. If you cannot get someone else to provide care, be careful to avoid the person you are caring for when you are coughing, sneezing, or blowing your

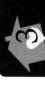

nose. Also, wash your hands after you cough, sneeze, or blow your nose. This will help prevent passing on the germs to him or her.

> ### Keep other people who have infections of any type away from the person with HIV/AIDS.

Decrease the number of visitors during the flu season. Remember that children acquire infections easily from schoolmates and can transmit them just as easily to the person with HIV/AIDS. Children with infectious conditions such as colds, chickenpox, and ear infections should be kept away from the person with HIV/AIDS or should be cared for in the home of a relative until they are well.

> ### Vaccinate against common problems.

Consider influenza and pneumococcal vaccinations for both the person you are caring for and for yourself. These vaccinations reduce the chance of catching the flu and pneumonia. (Consult with your doctor about these vaccinations because they can sometimes *cause* illness.)

> ### Wash hands often.

It is important that both you, the caregiver, and the person with HIV/AIDS wash your hands frequently to prevent infections. It is especially important that you wash your hands after using the toilet, after having your hands in soil, after handling pets or their toys, and before, as well as after, preparing food. Also, keep fingernails clean and do not bite them.

> ### Check with the doctor before having the children or adults in your home receive immunizations or booster shots.

Check with the doctor before having a child with HIV/AIDS receive immunizations or booster shots because these can sometimes cause illness. Also, check with the doctor before children or adults who live with a person with HIV/AIDS are vaccinated because they may "shed" vaccine strains of germs that could cause illness in the person with HIV/AIDS.

> ### Use plastic and washable toys for children with HIV/AIDS and their friends who visit.

> ### Encourage the person with HIV/AIDS to avoid using "recreational drugs" and having unprotected sex.

Needles, pipes, and other drug equipment can spread other infections to the person with HIV/AIDS, as can unprotected sex.

➤ **Discourage the person with HIV/AIDS from eating raw, unwashed fruits and vegetables, raw and undercooked meat, poultry, and fish, and from drinking unpasteurized milk.**

Bacteria found in raw and undercooked foods can cause various infections in the person with HIV/AIDS. Wash meat, poultry, and fish before cooking, and clean off surfaces that they have touched. (See also the home care plans "Opportunistic Infections" [Chapter 4] and "Fever and Infection" [Chapter 5].)

➤ **Have household pets cared for by persons other than the person with HIV/AIDS.**

Pet droppings contain high levels of bacteria and fungi that can be easily transmitted to the person you are caring for. (See also the home care plans "Opportunistic Infections" [Chapter 4] and "Fever and Infection" [Chapter 5].)

 POSSIBLE OBSTACLES TO CAREGIVING

Here are some attitudes, fears, and misconceptions that could prevent you from carrying out your plan:

"I can't take care of my son because I'm too afraid of getting AIDS from him."

Response: **The AIDS virus is not spread by caring for someone with HIV/AIDS.** Most often it is sexual contact or contact with the blood of a person with HIV/AIDS that spreads the virus. However, whether or not HIV/AIDS is transmitted through saliva is still unknown. Cooking, washing, cleaning, talking, touching, or helping the person with HIV/AIDS does not usually involve contact with blood or saliva, so these fears are usually unfounded.

"We've limited visitors in our home since my daughter came down with AIDS, because I would hate for a friend or neighbor to catch AIDS because of her illness."

Response: Visitors do not need to stay away and family members do not need to live in fear of contracting AIDS by simply being in the presence of someone who is HIV-positive or has AIDS. Have them read this chapter so that they understand how HIV/AIDS is spread.

Think of other obstacles

Identify additional roadblocks that could keep you from following the recommendations of this home care plan.

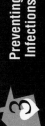

- Will the person I am caring for cooperate?

- Will other people help?

- How can I explain my needs to other people?

- Do I have the time and energy to carry out my plan?

You need to develop strategies for getting around roadblocks. Use the four COPE ideas (*C*reativity, *O*ptimism, *P*lanning, and *E*xpert information) to help you to develop new plans. See pp 4–8 for a discussion on how to use the four COPE ideas in overcoming your obstacles.

5. CARRYING OUT AND ADJUSTING YOUR PLAN

Checking on results

Review this chapter regularly to be sure that you are doing everything you can to prevent the spread of HIV/AIDS and the spread of other infections to the person you are caring for.

What to do if your plan does not work

1. Review this chapter.

2. If you find that you have skipped something, try it now.

3. Ask the doctor for further guidance if you continue to be worried about spreading infections or the HIV/AIDS virus.

4

Opportunistic Infections

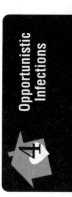

Overview of the Home Care Plan for *Opportunistic Infections*

 1. UNDERSTANDING THE PROBLEM

Causes of opportunistic infections

Effects of opportunistic infections on the person with HIV/AIDS

Your goals

 2. WHEN TO GET PROFESSIONAL HELP

Symptoms that indicate that professional help is needed

Information to have ready when you call

What to say when you call

 3. WHAT YOU CAN DO TO HELP

Supervise the use of antibiotics and medicines

Offer encouragement and reminders

 4. POSSIBLE OBSTACLES

 5. CARRYING OUT AND ADJUSTING YOUR PLAN

Carrying out your plan

Checking on results

What to do if your plan does not work

> **Topics that have an arrow (➤) in front of them are actions you can take or symptoms you can look for.**

Opportunistic Infections

1. UNDERSTANDING THE PROBLEM

Opportunistic infections occur when the immune system is not working properly. The infections occur in persons who have HIV/AIDS because they do not have the normal defenses to fight off organisms that cause infections. Opportunistic infections are more likely to occur when a special blood count, the CD4 or T_4 count, is below 200. The CD4 count for normal healthy adults is between 700 and 1200. For the person with HIV/AIDS, the CD4 count usually decreases gradually over time.

The organisms that cause opportunistic infections are categorized as protozoa, fungi, viruses, and bacteria. These organisms are found widely in nature and often live in the human body. Persons with defective immune system are unable to fight off the growth and destructive action of these organisms within the body. Opportunistic infections are seldom spread to people who have normal immune systems and are healthy.

> ➤ The information in this home care plan fits most situations, but yours may be different.
>
> ➤ If the doctor or nurse tells you to do something else, follow what he or she says.
>
> ➤ If you think there may be a medical emergency, see the section "When To Get Professional Help" on pp 42–44.

2. WHEN TO GET PROFESSIONAL HELP

Call the doctor or nurse if any of the following occur:

➤ **Changes in the person's mental functioning.**

This may or may not be accompanied by a stiff neck, a headache, or a fever. The person you are caring for will seem less alert, confused at times, forgetful, more irritable, or somewhat clumsy. These symptoms may point to an infection either within the brain or within the layers that cover the brain (called the *meninges*); the latter infection is called *meningitis*.

➤ **Coughing, difficulty breathing, or breathlessness, especially when moving.**

Pneumonia is a very common infection for persons with HIV/AIDS. Pneumonia can be treated, but treatment must begin early. A delay will result in breathing problems that are frightening, incapacitating, and possibly life-threatening. The person with HIV/AIDS is also very susceptible to tuberculosis, a respiratory infection that is easily spread even to healthy adults and children.

➤ **A long siege of diarrhea, lasting for 5 days or more, with six or more stools a day.**

Chronic diarrhea is often seen in persons with HIV/AIDS because the AIDS virus can affect the intestinal tract. Other organisms, such as salmonella, can also attack the digestive tract, causing symptoms such as abdominal cramping, uncontrolled diarrhea, and weakness. Although not all diarrhea is caused by opportunistic infections, it is important to report to health care professionals to determine the cause.

➤ **A painful rash, often seen on one side of the body, which seems to be spreading.**

Chickenpox and shingles (a painful rash) are caused by the herpes zoster virus. People with HIV/AIDS are vulnerable to this virus, and caregivers can also become infected if they come into contact with the weeping blisters. Those who have *not* had chickenpox are susceptible to both chickenpox and shingles because the same virus causes both conditions. Those caregivers who *have had* chickenpox cannot get it again. As always, a caregiver should use precautions to prevent contact with body fluids. (See the home care plan "Preventing the Spread of HIV and Other Infections" [Chapter 3].)

➤ Changes in vision.

Cytomegalovirus (CMV) infections, if left untreated, will result in blindness. The person with HIV/AIDS may complain of blurred vision, flashes of light, floating spots before the eyes, or blind areas within the visual field.

➤ Severe pain in the chest with swallowing.

Candida albicans is the fungus that causes thrush infections in the mouth and throat. It can also infect the esophagus, causing inflammation and pain each time the person swallows.

➤ Vaginal itching, irritation, and/or discharge develops.

Candida albicans often causes a yeast infection in the vagina of HIV-positive women that is difficult to get rid of.

When you call, have the answers ready to the following questions:

Problems involving the head

1. Has the behavior or alertness of the person you are caring for changed? When did this happen? Do either get worse at any particular time of the day?

2. Can the person tell you his or her name, the date, and where he or she is? Is he or she sleeping more?

3. Has he or she had any seizures?

4. Does he or she have any neck stiffness? If so, describe it.

5. Does he or she have headaches, and do they go away when treated with acetaminophen (e.g., Tylenol)?

6. Does a fever accompany any of the problems listed above?

Respiratory problems

7. Does the person you are caring for have a dry cough, or is he or she spitting up secretions? What color is the sputum?

8. Can he or she walk from one room to the next without feeling "breathless"?

9. How far (measured in feet) can he or she walk before feeling "breathless"?

10. Does he or she experience any chest pain when coughing, moving, or taking a deep breath?

11. Does a fever accompany the respiratory problems?

Gastrointestinal problems

12. Does the person you are caring for experience any nausea or vomiting?

13. Has he or she changed eating patterns or diet recently?

14. How does he or she feel after eating?

15. If he or she has diarrhea, when did it start? Describe the stool. How many stools are passed during a 24-hour period?

16. If he or she has diarrhea, what medicine is he or she taking to control it? Does it help? How often is it taken?

Skin problems

17. Does the person you are caring for have a new rash? Where is it located? How is this rash different from other rashes he or she has had in the past?

18. How does the rash feel (itches, burns, weeps, is hot)?

19. What medication is being applied to the rash? Does it help?

20. Does the person you are caring for experience any vaginal itching, irritation, or discharge?

Visual problems

21. How does the person you are caring for describe the eye problem?

22. Does he or she own prescription glasses, and if so, does he or she wear them? Does the vision improve when he or she wears the glasses?

23. Does the person complain of floating objects before the eyes? Can only one half of (actual) objects be seen?

It is important to know the person's CD4 count when describing symptoms. Symptoms become more of a concern when the CD4 count is low, for example, 20 as opposed to 500. Report the CD4 count along with the problems you are describing.

Here is an example of what you might say when calling for professional help:

"I am Rick Green, Bill Hoke's caregiver. Bill is a patient of Dr. Kroft. Bill says his eyes are blurry and he only sees half of what he's looking at. Bill's CD4 count, done 1 month ago, was 25."

 WHAT YOU CAN DO TO HELP

> **HERE ARE TWO STEPS YOU CAN TAKE:**
>
> Supervise the use of antibiotics and medicines
>
> Offer encouragement and reminders

Supervise the use of antibiotics and medicines

> ➤ **See that medications and antibiotics are taken at the prescribed times.**
>
> Because the person with HIV/AIDS often has many medications to take, some of which can cause nausea and other side effects, the person you are caring for may be tempted to omit medications or to stop taking them altogether. Help the person you are caring for to stick to medication schedules. Remind him that missing doses will make the medicines less effective.

> ➤ **Consider using medication boxes.**
>
> If the person you are caring for has difficulty remembering to take medicines, medication boxes (also called *compliance packs*) can be used. These plastic boxes, usually set up weekly, are divided into times of the day and days of the week. Using compliance packs is a way for the caregiver to verify whether the person has remembered to take medications at the prescribed times. If you can't find a plastic medicine box to suit your needs, an empty egg carton can work just as well; simply mark each slot with the name of the day of the week and the time that medicine is to be given that day.

> ➤ **Offer to assist with needed treatments.**
>
> Because certain treatments can be unpleasant (for example, pentamidine treatments administered monthly to prevent *Pneumocystis carinii* pneumonia), people with HIV/AIDS tend to omit them. Fatigue also interferes with how often the person with HIV/AIDS takes skin treatments and checks his or her temperature, and even how often he or she bathes and

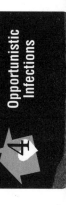

brushes teeth. Your assistance and encouragement are important. For example, you can put a checklist on the bathroom mirror or start a routine, such as brushing teeth after all meals.

Offer encouragement and reminders

➤ **Encourage but do not scold.**

Avoid preaching or scolding. These techniques are discouraging and offensive. Again, offering assistance and providing gentle reminders about the purpose and importance of certain treatments or medications is always more effective. Be creative. Assist the person you are caring for to manage treatments and medications himself or herself.

➤ **Encourage a healthy lifestyle.**

See that the immune system of the person you are caring for is supported through good nutrition, restful sleep, moderate exercise, good hygiene, stress management, and pleasurable experiences. Make sure that he or she avoids alcohol, "recreational drugs," tobacco, and "unsafe sex."

4. POSSIBLE OBSTACLES TO CAREGIVING

Here are some attitudes or misconceptions that could prevent you from carrying out your plan:

"This cough and headache are just from a cold I've picked up (or from my smoking). It should clear up in a few days if I take things easy."

Response: For a person with HIV/AIDS, a cough is often the first sign of a serious respiratory infection. If it is not treated quickly, it may become a life-threatening pneumonia that is much harder to treat. Smoking makes the cough and respiratory distress worse. Also, smoking promotes the progression of AIDS. Call health professionals about colds and headaches *early* rather than later.

"Headaches are a regular part of my life. When I get upset they come more often. This one will pass as soon as I relax."

Response: With HIV/AIDS, headaches that are persistent or hard to control or that cause changes in the person's ability to think may be a sign of a more serious problem that should not be ignored. Report such headaches, especially if the CD4 count is low or has not been measured recently.

Think of other obstacles

Identify additional roadblocks that could keep you from following the recommendations of this home care plan.

- Will the person I am caring for cooperate?

- Will other people help?

- How can I explain my needs to other people?

- Do I have the time and energy to carry out my plan?

You need to develop plans for getting around these roadblocks. Use the four COPE ideas (*Creativity, Optimism, Planning,* and *Expert information*) in developing your plans. See pp 4–8 for a discussion on how to use the four COPE ideas in overcoming your obstacles.

5. CARRYING OUT AND ADJUSTING YOUR PLAN

Carrying out your plan

Infections must be treated as soon as possible. In order to deal with opportunistic infections early, you must be alert for any changes in normal patterns. The body will give alerting signs that all is not well and that an infection is in progress.

Checking on results

If the person you are caring for is feeling better, you are making progress. Pay attention to which recommendations are working, and keep a "diary" of your progress. Continue to encourage him or her to keep taking the medications and treatments that will prevent further opportunistic infections.

What to do if your plan does not work

1. Review this chapter.

2. If you find that you've skipped something, try it now.

3. If you find that you've done all that you can, call the doctor for further guidance.

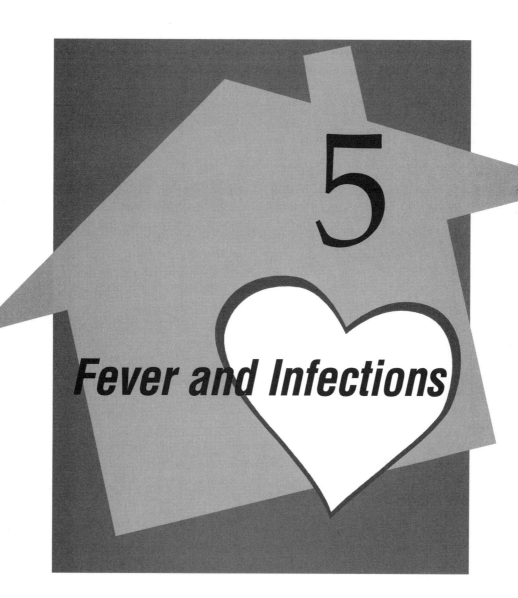

5

Fever and Infections

Overview of the Home Care Plan for
Fever and Infections

1. UNDERSTANDING THE PROBLEM

Infections and the person with HIV/AIDS

Signs of infection

Fever as one sign of infection

Your goals

2. WHEN TO GET PROFESSIONAL HELP

Symptoms that indicate an emergency

Symptoms that do not indicate an emergency but should be reported

Information to have ready when you call

What to say when you call

3. WHAT YOU CAN DO TO HELP

Reduce fever after reporting it

Prevent infections

4. POSSIBLE OBSTACLES TO CAREGIVING

5. CARRYING OUT AND ADJUSTING YOUR PLAN

Checking on results

What to do if your plan does not work

> **Topics that have an arrow (➤) in front of them are actions you can take or symptoms you can look for.**

Fever and Infections

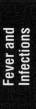

1. UNDERSTANDING THE PROBLEM

Fever, defined as a temperature higher than normal, is the most common sign of an infection. Other common signs of infection include fatigue, swelling, shaking chills, cough, pain, and headache. Chronic fevers are common with HIV/AIDS, but when a new fever is noticed in a person with HIV/AIDS, it should be checked out by a doctor. Thereafter, chronic fevers should be watched carefully. Fevers may become persistent as the disease progresses, and such fevers are very physically taxing. A new fever that is higher than usual (greater than 101 °F [38.3 °C]) can be a sign of a new infection requiring treatment with new or different antibiotics. Untreated fevers also add to weakness and fatigue.

Infections are caused by organisms or germs, such as bacteria, viruses, and fungi, that invade the body and begin to grow. Persons who are HIV-positive or who have developed AIDS are more likely to get infections because their immune systems are not working to protect them. The AIDS virus attacks the immune system and destroys it. When the CD4 count (T4 lymphocyte count) is 200 or less, the person is especially susceptible to infections.

> ➤ The information in this home care plan fits most situations, but yours may be different.
>
> ➤ If the doctor or nurse tells you to do something else, follow what he or she says.
>
> ➤ If you think there may be a medical emergency, see the section "When To Get Professional Help" on pp 52–55.

2. WHEN TO GET PROFESSIONAL HELP

Symptoms that indicate an emergency

Call the doctor, nurse, or the "after hours" phone number *immediately* if **any** of the following occurs:

➤ **A temperature that is 2 degrees higher than the person's normal temperature (after you have checked the temperature twice over a 2-hour period).**

Most normal oral temperatures are around 98.6 °F (37 °C) and can rise to 100.4 °F (38 °C) in the evening, but some people can have "normal" temperatures that are higher or lower than these. Consult with the doctor or nurse to learn beforehand (*before* an emergency occurs) what the normal temperature is of the person you are caring for. Bear in mind that a person with HIV/AIDS may have a chronic or persistent fever of 99 °F to 101 °F most of the time and that a normal temperature will usually rise in the late afternoon hours.

Check the temperature twice over a 2-hour period to be sure that there is a fever. You may want to buy a new thermometer if you have one that you do not trust or cannot read. A digital thermometer is the easiest to use and takes the guesswork out of taking a temperature: It lights up and shows you the exact temperature in digital numbers. Ask your pharmacist or a store clerk to help you select one.

➤ **A new fever when accompanied by any of the following symptoms:**

Headache

Stiff neck

Shortness of breath

Abdominal pain

Low back pain

Nausea/vomiting/diarrhea

Mental changes or confusion

Lightheadedness or dizziness with standing or sitting

Skin rash

➤ **Severe shaking chills that last 20 minutes or that come and go over a 1-hour period.**

Chills occur before a temperature goes up. Take the temperature after the chills and shaking have stopped unless they continue for more than 1 hour. Take a temperature *during* the chills if they last for more than 1 hour.

➤ **Frequent, painful urination.**

Painful urination indicates a urinary tract infection. Usually the person with this type of infection urinates in very small amounts. A person with a urinary tract infection feels a constant urge to pass urine even if little urine is in the bladder.

➤ **No urine output for 24 hours.**

It is very important to report if the person you are caring for has not urinated in the last day or has urinated very little. This condition has a variety of causes and needs to be investigated. It may be a sign of dehydration and may indicate the need for increased fluids, even intravenous (IV) fluids. It may also be a sign that the kidneys are not functioning properly.

➤ **New cough, shortness of breath, or rapid breathing.**

Report any problems with the respiratory tract, especially the feeling that it is hard to draw air into the lungs or release it. Labored or difficult breathing, with or without a fever, is important to report.

When symptoms are *not an emergency* but should be reported

Some symptoms that should be reported during regular office or clinic hours, even though they do not indicate an emergency, include the following:

➤ **The person you are caring for has a fever and is too weak to drink fluids.**

Report if the person you are caring for has a fever and is drinking very little. Drinking fluids is very important in a person with a fever because the body loses water when the body temperature rises. Dehydration may occur if the fever causes severe sweating and fluids are not being replaced.

➤ **Any redness or swelling near the site of a venous access device (for example, an IV, a Mediport, Hickman, Groshong, port-a-cath, or PICC Line).**

Venous access devices can become infected at any time after placement. This can happen even when great care has been taken to keep the site clean and free of contamination.

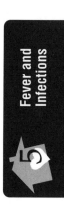

> **Any change in appearance of an open wound on the skin.**

Any open wound on the skin can become infected when the immune system is not working normally. The area may become more red and more tender. The wound may look deeper or the drainage from it may have changed color.

> **Cold symptoms, sore throat, or sinus pain or drainage.**

Infections can develop quickly in the mouth or throat. Report these symptoms even if they are not accompanied by fever.

> **Any change in menstrual pattern, such as a missed menstrual period or bleeding between periods.**

Menstrual abnormalities or irregularities have a variety of causes, including pregnancy, infection, tumors, and hormonal imbalances. Because the immune system of HIV-positive women is compromised, any potential sign of infection or cancer, such as a change in the menstrual pattern, should be reported.

> **Vaginal itching, irritation, or discharge.**

Women with HIV/AIDS women tend to have more gynecologic infections than other women. Vaginal candidiasis, also known as a yeast infection, is the most common. Symptoms included vaginal itching and a white curdlike discharge. This infection often persists in women with HIV/AIDS, despite the use of over-the-counter medicine, so report the symptoms.

> **Lower abdominal pain.**

In women with HIV/AIDS, lower abdominal pain may be a symptom of pelvic inflammatory disease (PID), a serious infection. This infection is equally likely in women with or without HIV/AIDS.

When you call, have the answers ready to the following questions:

1. For how many hours has the fever persisted (greater than 101 °F [38.3 °C] by mouth)?

2. Are the fevers sometimes less than 101 °F (38.3 °C)? If so, at what time of day?

3. How much liquid was taken over the last 8 hours?

4. Does the person you are caring for have an intravenous device, such as a Mediport, Hickman, Groshong, port-a-cath, or PICC Line?

5. Have any medicines been given to reduce fever or fight an infection (for example, acetaminophen, ibuprofen [Advil], or antibiotics)? If so, when?

6. Have you tried any other methods of reducing fever (i.e., not medication), such as sponge baths, fans, or cooling blankets?

7. Has the person you are caring for recently started taking any new medications? If so, what are they?

8. Were any blood counts measured recently, and if so, what were the test results?

9. For women, have there been any vaginal symptoms, lower abdominal pain, changes in menstrual flow or pattern of menstrual period?

Here is an example of what you might say when calling for professional help:

"I am Joan Smith, Alice Jones' caregiver. Joan is Dr. Black's patient. An hour ago, she had shaking chills that lasted for more than 20 minutes, and she had a temperature of 102.5 °F. Alice is also saying that she has a bad headache. What should I do? Do you think she has a new infection?"

3. WHAT YOU CAN DO TO HELP

> **HERE ARE TWO STEPS YOU CAN TAKE:**
>
> Reduce fever after reporting it
>
> Prevent infections

Reduce fever after reporting it

➤ **Give acetaminophen.**

Certain medicines (antipyretics), such as acetaminophen (e.g., Tylenol) or aspirin, reduce fevers. These drugs will not eliminate the cause of the fever, but they will make the person who is ill feel more comfortable. Give acetaminophen (2 tablets every 4 hours) for 24 hours, then stop. Check the temperature every 4 hours after this.

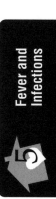

Fever and Infections

➤ **Make certain that all medications are taken that have been prescribed by the doctor for fever or infection.**

➤ **Apply cool washcloths to the forehead of the person you are caring for if he or she is uncomfortably hot.**

Cooling the forehead brings some relief from the discomfort of fever by cooling the blood that flows through the head close to the surface of the skin.

➤ **Change damp clothing and bed linens.**

If fever is accompanied by profuse sweating, the person you are caring for can get chills from the moisture. This adds to the discomfort brought on by the fever.

➤ **Encourage drinking plenty of fluids during a fever.**

Unless the doctor has instructed that fluids be restricted, encourage the person who has a fever to drink 2 to 3 quarts of cool fluids over a 12-hour period. During a fever, more fluids than usual are being lost through the skin and lungs, which may lead to dehydration. Drinking 2 to 3 quarts of fluids reduces this risk.

Prevent infections

➤ **If you have a cold, sore throat, or the flu, arrange for someone else to care for the person with HIV/AIDS until you are well.**

If you cannot find anyone to fill in for you, make certain that you wash your hands carefully before caring for the ill person.

➤ **Do not share personal items.**

It is especially important that anything that is used orally (for example, a thermometer or toothbrush) not be shared.

➤ **Ask people who have colds or who are ill to wait until they are better to visit.**

➤ **Maintain good personal hygiene.**

Hand washing is the best way to limit the spread of germs. Both the person with HIV/AIDS and those who come in contact with him or her should wash their hands frequently and brush their teeth at least twice daily to help kill the germs that cause infections. If this is a problem because areas of the skin or mouth are sore, read the home care plan "Problems with the Mouth" (Chapter 7).

➤ **Prevent infection caused by certain foods.**

Infections can be caused by unwashed raw fruits and vegetables; raw or poorly cooked eggs, fish, meat, and poultry; and unpasteurized milk. This is because of the bacteria and parasites that these foods carry. Proper washing and cooking will destroy sources of infection in food. Proper food storage is also important.

➤ **Encourage drinking plenty of fluids.**

Increased fluid intake will help prevent urinary infections. Urinary infections are less likely to occur when the kidneys, bladder, and urinary system are well flushed with plenty of fluids, especially water.

➤ **Encourage cleaning the rectal area thoroughly after bowel movements, especially if he or she has diarrhea.**

Women especially should cleanse the rectal area from front to back to reduce the likelihood of a urinary tract infection. Also, keeping the rectal area clean, particularly when diarrhea is a problem, will help keep the rectal area from getting raw or sore.

➤ **Consult with the health professional if you are planning to travel.**

You may need special immunizations and medicines to take with you.

➤ **Encourage wearing shoes or some other form of footwear to prevent cuts or sores on the feet.**

Make sure that shoes fit well and do not rub or cause blisters. Wash cuts or sores immediately with soap and water. Even small cuts or sore areas on the feet can let bacteria into the body.

➤ **Encourage using lotions and moisturizers on the skin to prevent drying, chapping, or cracking.**

Lotions boost the ability of the skin to stay intact by keeping the skin moist. Bacteria can enter dry skin cracks, leading to infection.

➤ **Encourage wearing gloves when working in soil.**

Soil has bacteria that can cause infection when in contact with skin cuts.

➤ **Arrange for someone other than the person with HIV/AIDS to groom the pet, empty cat litter boxes, and clean pet cages or fish tanks.**

Pet feces (stools) contain bacteria and fungi that can cause an infection in a person whose immune system is not functioning normally. If the person you are caring for is scratched or bitten by a pet, wash the site well and call the doctor or nurse if it begins to look infected. Stay up to date on routine vaccinations for your pets and tetanus boosters for yourself. Always wash your hands after handling pets, their toys, their hygiene items, their food and water, and their rugs and blankets. Be sure to have someone other than the person with HIV/AIDS wash fish tanks or reptile tanks.

POSSIBLE OBSTACLES TO CAREGIVING

Here are some common attitudes, fears, and misconceptions that may prevent you from carrying out your plan:

"High fevers can be controlled by Tylenol. I'll just take a few and not worry."

Response: High fevers, especially if they are new fevers, may indicate an infection. Taking a few acetaminophen tablets is *not* the only action needed. Careful monitoring of the fever and associated symptoms and reporting the temperature to the doctor or nurse is very important. This will ensure that treatment is started early, before the condition worsens.

"I've had fevers before, and they didn't last long. This one will go away like the others."

Response: Fevers can be the sign of a serious infection in the body. Remind the person you are caring for that fever needs to be reported, especially if it is new, so the infection can be treated.

Think of other obstacles

Identify additional roadblocks that could keep you from following the recommendations in this home care plan:

- Will the person with HIV/AIDS cooperate?

- Will other people help?

- How should I explain my needs to other people?

- Do I have the time and energy to carry out my plan?

You need to develop plans for getting around these roadblocks. Use the four COPE ideas (*C*reativity, *O*ptimism, *P*lanning, and *E*xpert information) in developing your plans. See pp 4–8 for a discussion on how to use the four COPE ideas in overcoming your obstacles.

5. CARRYING OUT AND ADJUSTING YOUR PLAN

Checking on results

Check on how effectively you are controlling fevers and preventing infections. Are fevers and infections occurring less often? Pay attention to which recommendations are working for you and which ones the person with HIV/AIDS is following. (For example, is the person with HIV/AIDS avoiding situations that increase the risk of his or her getting an infection?) Keep a "diary" of your progress.

What to do if your plan does not work

1. Review this chapter.

2. If you find that you've skipped something, try it now.

3. If you find that you've done all that you can, call the doctor for further guidance.

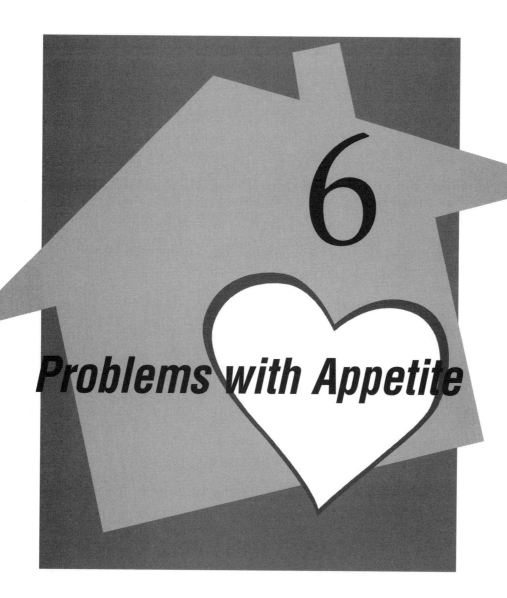

6

Problems with Appetite

Overview of the Home Care Plan for
Problems with Appetite

 1. **UNDERSTANDING THE PROBLEM**

   Causes of appetite problems

   Your goals

2. **WHEN TO GET PROFESSIONAL HELP**

   Symptoms indicating the need for professional help

   Information to have ready when you call

   What to say when you call

3. **WHAT YOU CAN DO TO HELP**

   Increase the appetite

   Cover up bothersome tastes and smells

   Prevent an early feeling of fullness

   Serve foods high in calories and protein

   Know the other options for boosting nutrition

 4. **POSSIBLE OBSTACLES TO CAREGIVING**

5. **CARRYING OUT AND ADJUSTING YOUR PLAN**

   Checking on results

   What to do if your plan does not work

> **Topics that have an arrow (➤) in front
> of them are actions you can take or
> symptoms you can look for.**

Problems with Appetite

1. UNDERSTANDING THE PROBLEM

People with HIV/AIDS commonly experience difficulty eating, poor appetite, and even complete loss of desire for food. Poor appetite can be caused by any of several factors, such as the disease itself; medications; soreness of the mouth, tongue, or throat; fatigue; and depression. For example, medicines used to treat HIV/AIDS can cause nausea, vomiting, diarrhea, and unpleasant changes in the taste of food and smell of food.

A sore mouth, tongue, or throat makes eating, chewing, and swallowing difficult, causing the ill person to avoid eating, even when he or she is hungry. The person with HIV/AIDS who suffers from fatigue, shortness of breath, fever, depression, or weakness may find it a chore to buy and prepare food and even to eat it. When loss of appetite leads to *weight loss*, health problems become even greater—particularly because good nutrition helps the body fight infection. Together, you and the person you are caring for can set several goals to solve this problem.

> ➤ The information in this home care plan fits most situations, but yours may be different.
>
> ➤ If the doctor or nurse tells you to do something else, follow what he or she says.
>
> ➤ If you think there may be a medical emergency, see the section "When To Get Professional Help" on pp 64–65.

2. WHEN TO GET PROFESSIONAL HELP

Call the doctor or nurse if any of the following occurs:

➤ **Very little intake of food or drink for 2 days or more.**

Report what you believe to be the cause of the loss of appetite—for example, nausea.

➤ **Rapid weight loss (at least 4 pounds lost during 1 week).**

Rapid weight loss causes a loss of energy and contributes to fatigue. Weight loss can be particularly rapid when there is significant diarrhea. If this is happening, it is important to alert a health professional.

➤ **Chewing or swallowing is painful.**

Painful chewing or swallowing interferes with normal eating and drinking. The pain may be caused by a mouth sore or an infection of the tongue, gums, or throat. If person you are caring for experiences a decrease in appetite, ask if he or she finds chewing or swallowing painful. After you report this to the doctor, medication may be prescribed to relieve mouth and throat pain.

When you call, have the answers ready to the following questions:

1. When did the appetite problem start?

2. If this problem has occurred before, what helped improve the appetite?

3. Is food less appealing because it tastes "different"—that is, bitter or metallic?

4. Is the person you are caring for able to drink fluids?

5. Is dryness or soreness of the mouth a problem, and has swallowing become difficult?

6. Do you have medication to help with mouth problems?

7. Does the person you are caring for feel full or bloated soon after starting to eat?

8. Is he or she experiencing nausea, vomiting, constipation, or diarrhea?

9. When the loss of appetite began, was there a significant decrease in the amount of food being eaten each day?

10. Are there certain meals or certain times of day when the appetite is better? Are there certain times when it is worse?

11. How much weight has been lost, and over what period of time?

12. Has he or she started any new medications recently?

13. Does he or she have a fever?

14. When eating, does he or she cough or does the voice sound "wet"?

15. Is there pain in areas other than the mouth or throat?

16. Is he or she depressed?

Here is an example of what you might say when calling for professional help:

"I am Henry Jones, Pete Walker's caregiver. Pete is a patient of Dr. Black. Pete says that he has almost no appetite at all. He also says that his food has developed a bitter taste and that this is causing him to avoid eating."

 3. **WHAT YOU CAN DO TO HELP**

HERE ARE FIVE STEPS YOU CAN TAKE:

Increase the appetite of the person you are caring for

Cover up bothersome tastes and smells

Prevent an early feeling of fullness

Serve foods high in calories and protein

Know the other options for boosting nutrition

Increase the appetite

Health professionals start with the easiest ways to improve appetite, such as smaller meals or ways to add protein and calories. They do not suggest tube feedings or intravenous (IV) feedings unless they are absolutely necessary.

➤ **Encourage light exercise or walking outdoors before meals.**

Any increase in activity just before eating increases the appetite. Try encouraging walking 5 to 15 minutes or even as long as 30 minutes before meals. Fresh air also often stimulates the appetite. However, the person you are caring for should avoid becoming overheated or overtired within a half an hour before a meal.

➤ **Serve meals with other people.**

Make eating a special activity. Eating with other people can increase the amount a person eats by taking attention away from food and by having mealtime a pleasurable experience and a time of companionship.

➤ **Serve meals in a pleasant, relaxed atmosphere.**

Noise, confusion, and loud music should not be permitted during mealtime.

➤ **Use small plates and serve smaller portions.**

Large portions can be discouraging to a person who is ill, and he or she may simply reject them altogether rather than try to eat even just a little bit. A small portion arranged attractively on a smaller-sized plate, on the other hand, appears "easy to eat."

➤ **Keep food out of sight when it is not mealtime.**

Place food in closed containers or in the refrigerator, and keep food off countertops. Seeing food at times other than mealtime may just remind the person you are caring for of his or her poor appetite.

➤ **Serve lemonade or orange juice.**

These juices contain acids that stimulate the appetite. Try serving about 4 ounces of any kind of tart-tasting juice. However, do not serve such juices if the person you are caring for has mouth sores.

➤ **Consult with a health professional or pharmacist about medication use.**

Changing the times that medication is taken or the dosage may help the appetite. Also, you might ask the doctor to prescribe antinausea medication or appetite stimulants.

Cover up bothersome tastes and smells

Treatments and medications frequently change how foods taste. Use the trial-and-error approach to find out which foods taste good and which do not. Taste change is often temporary and will probably disappear with time. If it returns later, however, you will have to use the trial-and-error approach again, because the foods that tasted good before may not be the same foods that taste good later.

➤ **Use plastic utensils.**

A bitter or "metallic" taste is a common side effect in people with HIV/AIDS. Using plastic forks, spoons, and knives help reduce this problem.

➤ **Try new spices.**

Spices make the mouth water and change the tastes of food. You may find a new spice that makes certain foods appealing again. Try cooking with basil, curry, coriander, mint, oregano, or rosemary. You should also try using old spices in new ways to change the way food tastes.

➤ **Add new flavors to foods to make them more appealing.**

Try cooking with lemon, beer, pickles, salad dressings, vinegar, vanilla, cinnamon, mayonnaise, relishes, fruit juices, and wines in creative ways.

➤ **Marinate meats.**

Marinate meats in fruit juices, salad dressings, wine, sweet and sour sauce, soy sauce, or barbecue sauce. Sauces and marinades change the flavors of foods and make them more appealing.

➤ **Sprinkle more sugar and salt on food if these are not restricted.**

Sugar and salt reduce "metallic" and bitter tastes.

➤ **Serve nutritious carbohydrates and high-protein foods.**

Foods such as fish, chicken, turkey, eggs, cheeses, milk, ice cream, tofu, nuts, peanut butter, yogurt, beans, and peas are high in carbohydrates and protein. Try to serve as much of these "power-packing" foods as possible.

➤ **Serve cold foods.**

Aromas are blocked or linger for shorter times when food is cold. Because cold foods are also sometimes less flavorful, "odd" or unpleasant tastes are not as noticeable. Also, the coolness some-

Appetite Problems

what "numbs" the tongue to some unappealing tastes. The food does not need to be frozen, just refrigerated.

➤ **Encourage the person you are caring for to suck on hard, sugar-free sour or mint candy.**

Candies such as these can mask strange tastes when eaten before a meal because their flavor stays in the mouth after they are eaten.

➤ **Serve ginger ale or mint tea.**

Ginger ale and mint tea cover up "metallic tastes" and help with swallowing food. When food tastes less metallic, the person is less likely to want to spit it out, and thus chewing and swallowing become easier.

➤ **Encourage the person you are caring for to avoid red meat.**

Changes in taste buds may make red meat distasteful. A person with HIV/AIDS may prefer chicken, fish, cheese, eggs, tofu, nuts, beans, and peas as sources of protein.

Prevent an early feeling of fullness

Poor appetite can be caused by an early feeling of "being full." Sometimes medicines cause gas and a feeling of bloating after even very little has been eaten. Here are some ways of preventing this feeling of fullness:

➤ **Exercise between meals.**

Any exercise stimulates the bowel muscles to move downward and shakes up pockets of gas. Stretching and bending at the waist, sometimes simply by rising from a chair or sofa, helps to relieve gas and to move and empty stomach contents. Walking or sitting up for a short time right *after* meals is also a good idea. However, strenuous exercise immediately after eating may cause cramps and should therefore be avoided.

➤ **Drink beverages *between* meals instead of *during* meals.**

Liquids at mealtime can make the stomach feel full. Drinking less while eating allows more room for food.

➤ **Eat small, frequent meals.**

Small, frequent meals or snacks eaten six to eight times a day prevent early fullness. Small meals are also easier to digest.

➤ **Eat slowly and chew food well.**

➤ **Cut back on fatty and gas-producing foods.**

Some vegetables naturally create stomach and intestinal gas and keep the person feeling full as the food is slowly digested. Foods such as beans, cucumbers, green peppers, onions, broccoli, Brussels sprouts, corn, cauliflower, sauerkraut, turnips, cabbage, chewing gum, milk, rutabaga, and carbonated beverages should be avoided. Remove the carbonation from beverages by opening cans and bottles early and letting the fizz evaporate.

➤ **Use over-the-counter medicines to help break up gas.**

One particular ingredient, simethicone, is very helpful in relieving gas and breaking up air trapped in the intestines. Check with the doctor, however, before buying these over-the-counter medicines because they should not be used with some other types of medicines.

Serve foods high in calories and protein

Rapid weight loss often can be slowed down by increasing the nutritional value of the food that is eaten, especially by serving foods high in calories and protein.

➤ **Offer small, frequent meals or snacks (six to eight per day), even if the person you are caring for is not hungry.**

Serving small, frequent meals and snacks will increase eating overall, which, in turn, will add up to higher protein and calorie intake. Encourage the person you are caring for to eat as much as possible.

➤ **Add butter or margarine to food.**

➤ **Add sugar, syrup, honey, and jelly to food.**

These toppings taste good when added to vegetables, cereals, waffles, and rolls.

➤ **Add whipped cream to hot chocolate, ice cream, pies, puddings, gelatin, and other desserts.**

➤ **Add milk, half and half, powdered coffee creamers, or powdered milk to gravy, sauces, soups, and hot cereals.**

These are also good sources of calcium.

➤ **Use milk instead of water to dilute condensed soups or cooked cereals.**

If a recipe calls for water, try using milk instead to add the extra calories.

> **Use mayonnaise instead of salad dressing, and use light cream instead of milk.**

Mayonnaise contains more fat than does salad dressing and is high in calories. Likewise, light cream has more fat and calories than does milk.

> **Add ice cream to milk drinks.**

Ice cream increases the fat and calorie content of the drink. Also, many people drink "Instant Breakfast" mixes for extra calories.

> **Add nonfat dry milk (1 cup) to one quart of whole milk for drinking and use in recipes.**

You can more than double the protein and calorie content of regular (4%) milk if you add powdered dry milk.

> **Serve snacks made with peanut butter.**

Peanut butter is an excellent source of protein and calories. It can be served on crackers, bread, waffles, apple wedges, and celery sticks.

> **Offer crushed granola, nuts, seeds, and wheat germ in shakes or on desserts.**

Serve these only when the mouth and throat are not too sore.

> **Add cheese to foods.**

Cheese is an excellent source of protein. Try adding it to eggs, meats, potatoes, vegetables, breads, salads, and soups.

Know the other options for boosting nutrition

> **Use liquid or powdered nutritional supplements in between meals or with snacks.**

These powders or liquids are loaded with nutrients and can be purchased in most drug stores. Ask the nurse or pharmacist for information about buying them, and ask them for recipes. Many people enjoy homemade milkshakes made with these supplements and ice cream.

> **Use vitamin supplements.**

Vitamin supplements, such as daily multivitamin and iron supplements, replace those vitamins that are lost because of poor appetite and decreased intake of food.

4. POSSIBLE OBSTACLES TO CAREGIVING

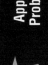

Here are some common attitudes, fears, and misconceptions that may prevent you from carrying out your plan:

"I find myself becoming frustrated and angry because the person I am caring for refuses to eat."

Response: When trying the recommendations given in this home care plan, do your best to be patient. Sometimes it takes much "trial-and-error" to learn what works best for increasing the appetite, and this may take more time than you had hoped. Meanwhile, don't focus on the appetite problem so much that it becomes the only topic you ask about or talk about.

"I'll start eating as soon as I start feeling better."

Response: If "feeling better" takes many days or even weeks, the person with HIV/AIDS can lose a great deal of weight and his or her appetite can completely disappear. Make certain that the person you are caring for understands this and that he or she must start trying *now* to increase intake of food.

Think of other obstacles

Identify additional roadblocks that could interfere with your following the recommendations in this home care plan:

- Will the person I am caring for cooperate?

- Will other people help?

- How can I explain my needs to others?

- Do I have the time and energy to carry out my plan?

You need to develop plans for getting around these roadblocks. Use the four COPE ideas (Creativity, Optimism, Planning, and Expert information). See pp 4–8 for a discussion of how to use the four COPE ideas in developing your plans.

5. CARRYING OUT AND ADJUSTING YOUR PLAN

Checking on results

Keep track of the amount of food the person with you are caring for is eating and check his or her weight regularly. Pay attention to which recommendations are working, and keep of "diary" of your progress.

What to do if your plan does not work

1. Review this chapter.

2. If you find that you've skipped something, try it now.

3. If you find that you've done all that you can, call the doctor for further guidance, especially if the person you are caring for is losing a great deal of weight and energy. The doctor may refer you to a dietitian who can give you new ideas and assess the diet with you.

A helpful booklet with tips for improving nutrition as well as the appetite is "Good Nutrition for People with HIV" (published by Channing L. Bete). Ask your nurse, nutritionist, or social worker to get you a copy. You may order it yourself by calling 1-800-628-7733.

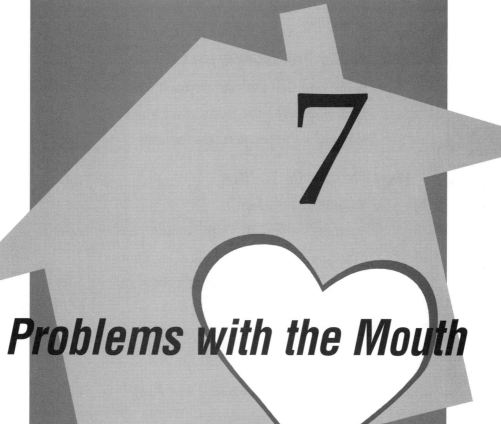

7

Problems with the Mouth

Overview of the Home Care Plan for
Problems with the Mouth

1. *Understanding the Problem*

> Causes of mouth sores and fungal infections in people with HIV/AIDS
>
> Your goals

2. *When To Get Professional Help*

> Symptoms that indicate the need for professional help
>
> Information to have ready when you call
>
> What to say when you call

3. *What You Can Do To Help*

> Keep the mouth moist
>
> Soothe a sore mouth or throat and ease swallowing
>
> Treat mouth sores, ulcers, and infections
>
> Prevent mouth sores and infections

4. *Possible Obstacles*

5. *Carrying Out and Adjusting Your Plan*

> Carrying out your plan
>
> Checking on results
>
> What to do if your plan does not work

**Topics that have an arrow (➤) in front
of them are actions you can take or
symptoms you can look for.**

Problems with the Mouth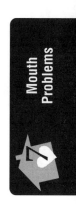

 ## UNDERSTANDING THE PROBLEM

Mouth sores or infections are common in people with HIV/AIDS. A yeast infection of the mouth caused by the fungus *Candida albicans* is known as *thrush*. Mouth problems may also be caused by viruses or by the medications used to treat HIV/AIDS.

When the immune system begins to fail because of the AIDS virus, mouth and throat problems can develop easily. Mouth discomfort and painful swallowing may cause the person with HIV/AIDS to avoid eating, which, in turn, leads to weight loss and weakness.

Often, persons who have yeast infections in the mouth and throat will need daily medications to treat the infection and to keep it from recurring. Although such infections can be controlled, they cannot be cured completely.

Other kinds of mouth problems include cavities and sore gums. These can be caused by inadequate brushing or flossing.

> ➤ The information in this home care plan fits most situations, but yours may be different.
>
> ➤ If the doctor or nurse tells you to do something else, follow what he or she says.
>
> ➤ If you think there may be a medical emergency, see the section "When To Get Professional Help" on p 76–77.

Mouth problems can sometimes become so severe that the person requires hospitalization for antibiotic therapy or intravenous feedings.

YOUR GOALS

Know when to seek professional help

Keep the mouth moist

Soothe a sore mouth or throat and ease swallowing

Treat mouth sores and infections

Prevent mouth sores and infections

---

2. WHEN TO GET PROFESSIONAL HELP

Call the doctor or nurse if any of the following occurs:

➤ **A sore mouth with a new temperature of more than 101 °F (38.3 °C) or 2 degrees above the person's normal temperature.**

Fever may accompany a mouth infection. If the temperature of the person you are caring for rises suddenly, report it to a health care professional. However, a mouth infection can occur even without fever, and a fever may indicate an infection other than a mouth infection.

➤ **The tongue becomes more reddened or new white patches appear on it.**

New white patches can appear on the gums and in the mouth as well. These indicate an infection. Usually it is a thrush infection (*Candida albicans*).

➤ **A sore or ulcer appears on the lips or in the mouth.**

Such sores may have many different causes and treatments. They should be reported immediately so that treatment may begin as soon as possible. Mouth sores caused by viral infections (canker sores, fever blisters) can be quite painful.

➤ **A sore throat.**

The lining of the throat is the same as the lining of the mouth, and is just as likely to get red and sore.

➤ **The person you are caring for is *not taking medicine as prescribed* because swallowing has become too painful.**

➤ **The person you are caring for *has eaten and drunk very little for more than 1 day* because swallowing has become too painful.**

Two days without nutrition or fluid will cause weakness and, possibly, dehydration.

➤ **Increased redness or bleeding of the gums.**

Sometimes people with HIV/AIDS do not take care of their teeth and do not floss or brush often enough because they are too tired or because they just never got into the habit of brushing often. The gums may become sore and painful abscesses or ulcers may develop, leading to infection or further problems.

When you call, have the answers ready to the following questions:

1. When did the mouth problems start?

2. What is the appearance of the mouth?

3. Is the person you are caring for able to eat or drink? If so, how much has he or she eaten and drunk during the past two days?

4. Has he or she noticed that hot, cold, or spicy foods make the mouth or teeth feel different?

5. When he or she swallows, how far down in the chest does the pain extend, and is the pain accompanied by a feeling that food is caught in the throat or esophagus (the swallowing tube from the throat to the stomach)?

6. Does he or she smoke or drink alcoholic beverages? If so, how much? Has his or her smoking and drinking increased?

7. Has he or she ever had mouth problems before now? If so, has he or she ever had this *same* problem?

8. What medications is the person you are caring for currently taking?

9. Is anything being done to reduce mouth or throat soreness? If so, how well is this treatment working?

Here is an example of what you might say when calling for professional help:

"I am Joan Smith, Harry Smith's caregiver. Harry is Dr. Brown's patient. Harry is complaining of a sore mouth and throat. There are white patches on his tongue and gums. Harry says that his throat is so sore that he can't eat or take his medicines."

3. WHAT YOU CAN DO TO HELP

HERE ARE FOUR STEPS YOU CAN TAKE:

Keep the mouth moist

Soothe a sore mouth or throat and ease swallowing

Treat mouth sores and infections

Prevent mouth sores and infections

Because mouth discomfort may cause the person you are caring for to drink less fluid, dry mouth may accompany his or her sore mouth and throat. Several steps can be taken to moisten a dry mouth:

➤ **Rinse the mouth with water before meals and throughout the day.**

Rinsing the mouth helps to moisten it and remove the feeling of being parched or dry.

➤ **Use a lip moisturizer before eating.**

If the lips are moist, food is easier to chew and enjoy. Petroleum jelly, lip salve, or cocoa butter can be used as lip moisturizers.

➤ **Sip 2 to 3 quarts of liquid per day, unless the person you are caring for has been restricted from drinking large amounts of fluid.**

If swallowing is painful, taking small sips may help ensure that the person you are caring for is receiving the proper amount of fluid each day. He or she should especially make an effort to take small sips of liquids with meals. Although it is important to drink plenty of water, fluids such as milk and juice provide more calories and nutrients.

➤ **Eat ice chips, Popsicles, and frozen juices.**

Ice chips and Popsicles are a refreshing source of fluids that do not need to be drunk. Popsicles also cause salivation, which decreases dryness.

➤ **Dunk bread, crackers, and baked foods into coffee, tea, milk, or soup to make them moist.**

➤ **Mix gravies, sauces, salad dressings, melted butter or margarine, mayonnaise, and yogurt into food.**

Sauces and gravies go a long way to moisten food and make it easier to chew and swallow. These can be added toward the end of cooking or when food is reheated.

➤ **Serve foods that are high in liquid content and are soft.**

Soft foods and foods that are high in liquid content include apple sauce, canned fruits, casseroles, cooked cereal, baby foods, Popsicles, custard, bananas, puddings, ice cream, gelatin, sherbet, yogurt, milkshakes, soups, stews, watermelon, and seedless grapes. Also, blenderizing foods can make foods easier to chew.

➤ **Use artificial saliva.**

Bottles of artificial saliva can be ordered through most pharmacies. It is made of glycerin, purified water, and a few other ingredients. Xero-Lube and Salivart are two commercial products that are available in mint flavor. Many people have found these products helpful in alleviating dry mouth.

Soothe a sore mouth or throat and ease swallowing

Here are some ways of soothing a sore mouth or throat:

➤ **After eating, rinse the mouth with a solution of 1/2 teaspoon of baking soda in one cup of tap water.**

Baking soda soothes the mouth and helps it heal, while rinsing the mouth after eating removes food particles that may irritate the gums. The baking soda solution is much more gentle than commercial mouthwashes, many of which contain alcohol. These should be avoided because they dry out the mouth.

➤ **Drink plenty of liquids and suck on ice chips.**

➤ **Serve soft foods.**

Soft foods are easier to chew and swallow, and they are less likely to make sores or scrape raw tissues. Some examples of such foods are soups, eggs, pancakes, pastas, quiches, baby foods, cheese dishes, tuna fish, apple sauce, custards, pudding, canned fruit, cooked cereals, bananas, gelatin, yogurt, ice cream, sherbet, frozen fruit bars, Popsicles, and milkshakes. It also a good idea to serve bland foods (foods that are not spicy or salty) because these foods are less likely to irritate the tissue of the mouth. Examples are bread, pudding, gelatin, custard, rice, and tapioca. You might try using a blender or hand masher to soften "harder" foods, or you could try moistening food with cream, milk, gravy, or sauces.

Foods to avoid: vegetables high in acidic content (for example, tomatoes) and soups and sauces made from these vegetables, potato skins, crunchy and raw vegetables, fried foods, citrus fruits (such as oranges, grapefruits, and lemons), seeded breads, crusty breads, and granola bars.

➤ **Serve foods at room temperature.**

Avoid *extremely* hot foods such as hot pizza.

➤ **Let carbonation, or fizz, escape from sodas.**

Carbonated beverages can irritate mouth sores and cause a burning sensation.

➤ **Serve high-calorie liquids, food supplements such as Ensure, and milkshake recipes.**

With these, the person gets the most calories with the least eating.

➤ **Avoid cigarettes, pipes, chewing tobacco, and alcoholic beverages.**

These will irritate mouth sores.

➤ **Serve pureed food from a cup or with a short straw.**

Soft food can be liquefied and poured into a cup for drinking. Using a short straw offers the additional advantage of bypassing some of the sore mouth tissue during eating and decreases the chance of taking in too much air, which causes gas. Also, shorter straws are easier to use and require less use of energy. Many proteins can be taken in this way. If the person you are caring for is too weak to use a straw himself or herself, help give fluids using a straw: First, dip the straw into the glass and hold your finger over the end of the straw. This will hold liquid in the straw. You can drip the liquid into the person's mouth by releasing the finger quickly and then covering it again. Fill the straw with only a very small amount of liquid, to avoid releasing too much into the mouth of the person who is ill. Practice this before actually trying to give liquids this way.

Treat mouth sores and infections

Try the following suggestions at the first sign of a sore or mouth infection. These may reduce the seriousness of mouth and throat complications.

➤ **Rinse with warm tap water or any of one of the following after eating and drinking:**

1/2 teaspoon salt in 2 cups of water, *or*

1/2 teaspoon baking soda in 1 cup of water, *or*

1/2 teaspoon salt and 1/2 teaspoon baking soda in 2 cups of water.

The person you are caring for should rinse his or her mouth frequently—at least four times per day and, while awake, as often as every 2 hours. Mouth rinses remove food particles that may build up and cause bacteria to grow. Rinses also soothe sore tissues and help them heal faster. If the salt rinse "burns," use less salt or use the baking soda solution.

➤ **Use a numbing medicine or mouth gels as a "throat coat" before eating and swallowing.**

Rinsing with or swallowing mouth gels that contain a numbing medicine (Viscous Lidocaine) before meals and whenever the mouth is very sore is helpful. This numbs the tongue and throat temporarily, allowing liquids and soft foods to be taken without too much trouble. Another type of soothing medicine (called a "slurry") comes in tablet form and is dissolved in water. It works quickly to remove any burning feeling and helps to heal the lining of the mouth and throat.

If the person you are caring for has trouble swallowing liquid medicines like these or does not use them as often as prescribed, tell the doctor so he or she can order another type of mouth treatment.

➤ **Use prescription mouth rinses to swish and swallow.**

Specially prepared mouth solutions containing Maalox, liquid Benadryl, and numbing medicine (Lidocaine) can soothe soreness, reduce swelling, and reduce inflammation in the mouth, throat, and esophagus. These mouth rinses will be ordered to be used at least every 4 to 6 hours.

➤ **Use antifungal medicines.**

These preparations come in the form of a liquid that is swished in the mouth and then swallowed (Nystatin swish and swallow solution), pills, or in the form of tablets and lozenges (Mycelex lozenges) that dissolve in the mouth much like a piece of hard candy. *These medicines treat the source of the infection.* They are ordered to be used between every 2 to 8 hours.

➤ **Use mild pain medication, if it is necessary.**

Mild pain pills may be taken 1 hour before eating and drinking. This will help to take the edge off of the discomfort felt when biting, chewing, and swallowing.

➤ **Avoid the use of hydrogen peroxide or peroxide rinses.**

While peroxide kills bacteria, it is very drying. Use peroxide only if recommended by your doctor.

Prevent mouth sores and infections

Here are several ways of preventing mouth problems:

➤ **See a dentist regularly, especially one who has helped others with HIV/AIDS.**

The dentist will clean the mouth, refit dentures if necessary, and spot mouth problems early, before they become severe.

➤ **Keep the mouth, teeth, and gums clean.**

After each meal, the person you are caring for should rinse his or her mouth with salt water or a baking soda solution (see p 81 for possible mixtures), as well as rinse with warm water several times during the day. Rinsing, even with just warm water, removes bacteria and food build-up that can lead to mouth infections and sores. *To be effective, mouth rinsing should be performed for at least 5 minutes.*

Dentures (partial or full) should be removed before rinsing the mouth. Food particles can easily collect under dentures, causing sores. This is even more likely when dentures are loose, which is frequently a result of weight loss. It is also important to keep dentures and partials clean.

To clean the teeth, use any of the following: (1) a soft-bristle toothbrush, (2) a soft-sponge applicator, (3) a cotton-tipped applicator, or (4) gauze or a soft washcloth. These prevent cutting or scraping and reduce the likelihood of infection.

Using dental floss at least once daily is another way of keeping the teeth and gums clean. Flossing removes food particles that become lodged between teeth.

➤ **Keep the lips moist.**

When swallowing is difficult, the mouth and lips become very dry. Lip balms, petroleum jelly, or cocoa butter can help prevent dryness and cracking.

➤ **Keep the mouth tissues moist.**

Encourage the person you are caring for to drink about 2 to 3 quarts of fluid each day, unless the doctor has ordered otherwise.

Drinking fluids washes out the mouth and helps keep sensitive tissues moist, which also can prevent infection.

Chewing sugarless gum or sucking on sugarless hard candies increases saliva in the mouth. Sugarless products are recommended because they limit the build-up of bacteria.

Commercial mouthwashes should be avoided. Many commercial mouthwashes contain alcohol, which will dry the mouth.

 4. **POSSIBLE OBSTACLES TO CAREGIVING**

Here are some common attitudes, fears, and misconceptions that may prevent you from carrying out your plan:

"It takes too much time to do all of that mouth rinsing. Besides, I forget to do it."

Response: Often the person you are caring for will fail to cooperate with the recommendations of the home care plan, or will underestimate the importance of the treatments. Try your best to make him or her understand the importance of good oral hygiene and to remind him or her to perform mouth rinses. Praise any attempts to care for the mouth and encourage this behavior.

"I don't want to quit smoking and drinking."

Response: If the person you caring for refuses to quit either habit, try to encourage him or her to "cut back." Also, if the person is a smoker, he or she should make an even greater effort to follow the other recommendations discussed in this chapter.

"Soft or mashed foods are unappetizing. They just remind me that I am sick."

Response: Serve soft foods attractively. Add flavorings to improve the taste of the foods. See the home care plan "Problems with Appetite" (Chapter 6) for suggestions on how to prepare foods in appealing ways.

Think of other obstacles

Identify additional roadblocks that could keep you from following the recommendations in this home care plan:

• Will the person I am caring for cooperate?

- Will other people help?

- How can I explain my needs to others?

- Do I have the time and energy to carry out this plan?

You need to develop plans for getting around these roadblocks. Use the four COPE ideas (*C*reativity, *O*ptimism, *P*lanning, and *E*xpert information) in developing your plans. See pp 4–8 for a discussion of how to use the four COPE ideas in overcoming your obstacles.

CARRYING OUT AND ADJUSTING YOUR PLAN

Carrying out your plan

Setting up and following a regular, daily routine for treating and preventing mouth sores and infections is the most important part of your plan. Make certain that the daily routine combines a regimen of oral hygiene and appropriate diet, as discussed in this chapter.

Checking on results

Take note of which recommendations are working, and keep a "diary" of your progress. Also, pay attention to whether any mouth problems are interfering with eating, to avoid the further complications, such as weight loss and physical weakness.

What to do if your plan does not work

1. Review this chapter.

2. If you find that you've skipped something, try it now.

3. If you find that you've done all that you can, call the doctor for further guidance.

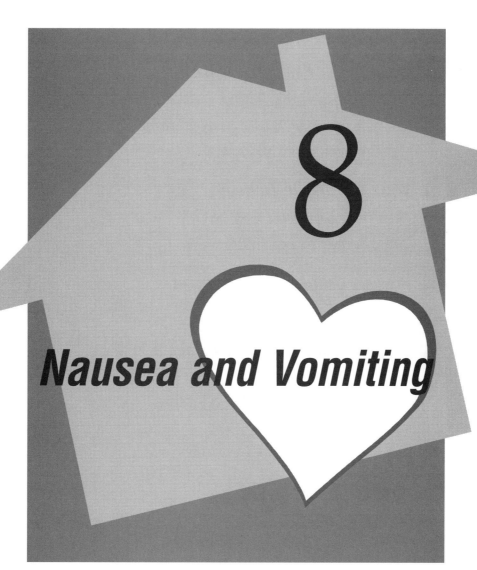

Nausea and Vomiting

8

Overview of the Home Care Plan for
Nausea and Vomiting

1. UNDERSTANDING THE PROBLEM

   Causes of nausea and vomiting in persons with HIV/AIDS

   Your goals

2. WHEN TO GET PROFESSIONAL HELP

   Symptoms that indicate an emergency

   Information to have ready when you call

   What to say when you call

3. WHAT YOU CAN DO TO HELP

   Use anti-nausea medicine

   Reduce nausea and vomiting

4. POSSIBLE OBSTACLES TO CAREGIVING

5. CARRYING OUT AND ADJUSTING YOUR PLAN

   Checking on results

   What to do if your plan does not work

> **Topics that have an arrow (➤) in front of them are actions you can take or symptoms you can look for.**

Nausea and Vomiting

1. UNDERSTANDING THE PROBLEM

Many of the medications used to fight infection and to limit the activity of HIV may cause nausea and vomiting in some people. Persons who develop AIDS-related cancer such as Kaposi's sarcoma may also experience some nausea or vomiting as a side effect of the chemotherapy and/or radiotherapy used to treat the cancer.

Nausea and vomiting should be controlled not only because these symptoms are uncomfortable but because they can lead to dehydration (lack of the proper amount of fluid in the body), increased fatigue, and decreased intake of food (which, in turn, may lead to weight loss).

> ➤ The information in this home care plan fits most situations, but yours may be different.
>
> ➤ If the doctor or nurse tells you to do something else, follow what he or she says.
>
> ➤ If you think there may be a medical emergency, see the section "When To Get Professional Help" on pp 88–90.

WHEN TO GET PROFESSIONAL HELP

Symptoms that indicate an emergency

Call the doctor, nurse, or "after hours" phone number *immediately* if any of the following occurs:

➤ **There is blood or material that looks like coffee grounds in the vomit.**

Vomit that looks like coffee grounds is really old blood and signals that some bleeding has occurred in the stomach. This should be reported *immediately*.

➤ **Vomiting that occurs more than once during a 24-hour period.**

Frequent vomiting can lead to dehydration. Report it immediately if the person vomits a second time less than 24 hours after the first time.

➤ **Projectile vomiting (the vomit shoots out at a distance).**

Projectile vomiting may indicate problems in the stomach or intestine, such as an obstruction, or it may indicate increased pressure inside the head. These conditions should be investigated by a doctor immediately.

➤ **Prescribed medicines cannot be "kept down" because of vomiting.**

Medicines should never be omitted. If the person you are caring for has missed as many as *two doses* because of nausea, contact a doctor immediately. He or she may prescribe different medication that can be tolerated (for example, in forms other than tablets). The doctor may also prescribe anti-nausea medicine, which is taken 30 minutes before the regular medication time to help "keep down" the medications.

➤ **The person you are caring for has had less than 8 ounces of liquid and/or has not eaten any solid food during a 24-hour period.**

To avoid dehydration, especially after continued vomiting, most people need to drink more than 6 cups of fluid during a 24-hour period. Also, going for 2 days without solid food is dangerous in most cases because the blood sugar will drop, particularly in persons who have a fever, which can increase dehydration. However, because each person's needs are different, ask your doctor when you should call.

➤ **Weakness or dizziness accompanies the nausea or vomiting.**

It is normal for a *little* weakness or dizziness to accompany nausea or vomiting, but if the person you are caring for can't even rise from a chair because of weakness or dizziness, you should contact the doctor immediately.

➤ **Severe stomach pain accompanies vomiting.**

Severe pain is always a reason to call the doctor immediately. It may indicate a stomach obstruction.

When you call, have the answers to the following questions ready:

1. How long has the person you are caring for been experiencing nausea or vomiting?

2. When does the nausea or vomiting begin and how long does it last?

3. How bad was the most recent attack of nausea or vomiting?

4. How much does the nausea interfere with normal activities?

5. Was medicine prescribed for nausea? (Include over-the-counter products the person you are caring for is currently using.)

   If so, what are the medicine(s)?

   How often should it (they) be taken?

   What dosage is prescribed? (For example, how many pills should be taken at one time, and how often?)

   How much of the medication has been taken during the last 2 days?

   How much relief has the medication given?

   How long has the relief tended to last?

6. What other means (other than anti-nausea medicine) have been tried to help the person with nausea to feel better? What have the results been?

7. Is the nausea ever followed by vomiting?

8. What does the vomit look like? Is this vomit different in color from earlier vomit? If so, how is it different?

9. How often has vomiting occurred during the past 24 hours?

10. What and how much has the person you are caring for eaten during the past 24 hours?

11. What and how much has the person you are caring for drunk during the past 24 hours?

12. How frequent have bowel movements been during the past 2 days? Have the stools been the same in amount and color?

13. Is the nausea accompanied by fever?

15. What other new symptoms have occurred since the nausea and/or vomiting began? (Answer questions below for each new symptom.)

SYMPTOM:_____ Where_____

How bad_____

When did it start_____

When does it happen_____ How long does it last_____

What relieves it_____

What does not help_____

Here is an example of what you might say when calling for professional help:

"I am Joan Smith, Harry Smith's caregiver. Harry is a patient of Dr. Jones. Harry has been having nausea and vomiting for more than a day now. Since last night, he hasn't been able to 'keep down' any food or medicine, not even water. He has missed two doses of his pain medicine."

 3. WHAT YOU CAN DO TO HELP

> **HERE ARE TWO STEPS YOU CAN TAKE:**
>
> Use anti-nausea medicine
>
> Reduce nausea and vomiting

Use anti-nausea medicine

Here are ways of using anti-nausea medicine effectively:

➤ **Take anti-nausea medicine on a consistent schedule, especially when nausea is a chronic problem.**

The person you are caring for should continue taking the medication for as long as the nausea persists. The anti-nausea medicine must be taken on a consistent schedule to maintain an adequate drug concentration in the blood.

➤ **Take anti-nausea medicines one half-hour before meals.**

One half-hour is generally the amount of time needed for the anti-nausea medicine to enter the system and reduce nausea.

➤ **Take anti-nausea medicine as prescribed by the doctor, usually before and after receiving chemotherapy or other treatments, and before taking medications that cause nausea and vomiting.**

As in the case of meals, the person you are caring for should take anti-nausea medicines about one half-hour before he or she takes medications that tend to cause nausea, as well as before scheduled treatments that cause nausea, such as chemotherapy. He or she should continue taking the anti-nausea medicine every 4 to 6 hours until the nausea is completely gone.

Reduce nausea and vomiting

Here are ways of reducing nausea and vomiting without the use of anti-nausea medications. *Start with those suggestions that have helped in the past, then move on to the ideas that are new to you.*

➤ **Avoid fried foods, dairy products, and acidic foods such as fruit juices or vinegar salad dressings.**

Fats are difficult to digest, and citrus juices may irritate the bowel. If fat intolerance is a problem, you may want to substitute medium-chain triglycerides (MCT) oil for regular cooking oil in recipes and use nutritional supplements that contain MCT oil (Lipisorb, Osmolite, Nutren, and Peptamen).

➤ **Use chewing gum, hard candy, and oral "rinses" to freshen the mouth.**

Try peppermint or fruit-flavored gum and candy. These will cover up any unpleasant or bitter taste in the mouth. However, remember that chewing gum can produce stomach gas

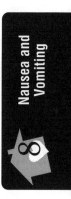

Nausea and Vomiting

8

so don't encourage the person with HIV/AIDS to chew it all day.

➤ **Let fresh air into the house, or encourage the person you are caring for to spend some time outside.**

Taking in fresh air helps relieve the feeling of nausea. Also, suggest mouth breathing for a few minutes to get more air and see if the nausea is relieved.

➤ **Rest.**

Some people find it helpful to lie down when they are nauseated. Anti-nausea medicine will often make people sleepy, which helps them to sleep through their nausea and relieve it.

➤ **Drink fluids 2 hours after vomiting.**

After the vomiting has passed, the person you are caring for should wait a while (about 2 hours) before trying to eat or drink. He or she should take no more than 1 to 2 ounces at a time. Also, the person you are caring for should let the fizz go out of soda before drinking it because carbonation (bubbles) may upset the stomach again. Pour the soda into a glass and stir vigorously with a spoon to release carbonation and bubbles.

➤ **Eat dry crackers.**

Eating dry crackers, a method often used by pregnant women to decrease nausea, can also help the person with HIV/AIDS.

➤ **Eat 3 to 4 hours before treatments, and eat frequently at other times.**

Encourage the person you are caring for to eat 3 to 4 hours before treatments that cause nausea. This ensures that the stomach is not completely empty at the time of the treatment and that the body is being supplied with needed nutrition during the treatment. Eating frequent light meals throughout the day is another way of fighting nausea.

➤ **Avoid unpleasant or strong odors.**

Encourage the person you are caring for to stay away from rooms such as the kitchen if they have heavy odors. Breathing through the mouth may also prevent nausea caused by odors, including odor from cigarette smoke, air fresheners, heavy perfumes, or aftershave lotions.

➤ **Wear loosely fitting clothes.**

The person you are caring for should avoid tight-fitting material, especially around the waist or neck. These items put pressure on the throat and stomach, adding to the feeling of nausea.

➤ **Become involved in pleasant distractions.**

Pleasant distractions that do not require much physical exertion, such as watching television or reading, may help take the focus off of the nausea. Relaxation techniques, such as listening to soothing music, thinking about peaceful scenes or images, or receiving a massage may also help.

 ## 4. POSSIBLE OBSTACLES TO CAREGIVING

"I'll simply have to get used to the nausea caused by my medications. After all, most medicines that are strong enough to treat a disease should cause nausea and vomiting."

Response: Nausea can and should be controlled. If a medicine is causing nausea and vomiting, ask your doctor to recommend anti-nausea medicines.

Think of other obstacles

Identify additional roadblocks that could keep you from following the recommendations in this home care plan:

- Will the person I am caring for cooperate?
- Will other people help?
- How can I explain my needs to others?
- Do I have the time and energy to carry out this plan?

You need to develop plans for getting around these roadblocks. Use the four COPE ideas (Creativity, Optimism, Planning, and Expert information) in developing your plans. See pp 4–8 for a discussion of how to use the four COPE ideas in overcoming your obstacles.

 ## 5. CARRYING OUT AND ADJUSTING YOUR PLAN

Checking on results

You can check on how well this home care plan is working by keeping track of how often vomiting and nausea are occurring, how severe the feelings of nausea are, and how much nausea is causing the person you are caring for has cut back on normal activities. Pay attention to which recommendations are working, and keep a "diary" of your progress..

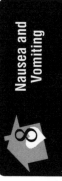

What to do if your plan does not work

1. Review this chapter.

2. If you find that you've skipped something, try it now.

3. If you find that you've done all that you can, call the doctor for further guidance.

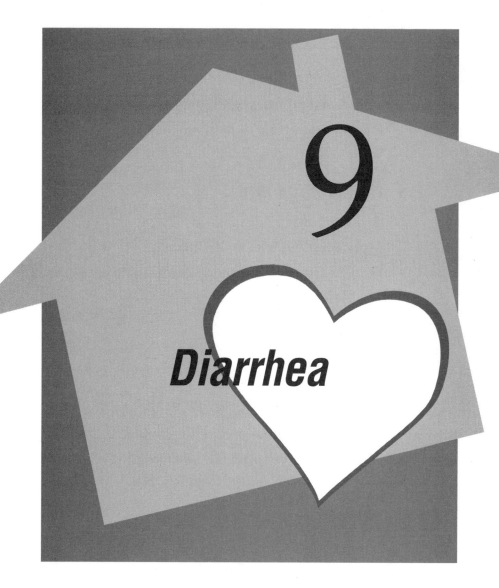

9

Diarrhea

Overview of the Home Care Plan for
Diarrhea

 1. UNDERSTANDING THE PROBLEM

Causes of diarrhea in people with HIV/AIDS

Your goals

 2. WHEN TO GET PROFESSIONAL HELP

Symptoms that indicate an emergency

Information to have ready when you call

What to say when you call

 3. WHAT YOU CAN DO TO HELP

Give medicines for diarrhea

Replace lost fluids and nutrients

Encourage the person you are caring for to avoid certain foods

Increase comfort and protect the skin

4. POSSIBLE OBSTACLES

 5. CARRYING OUT AND ADJUSTING YOUR PLAN

Checking on results

What to do if your plan does not work

Topics that have an arrow (➤) in front of them are actions you can take or symptoms you can look for.

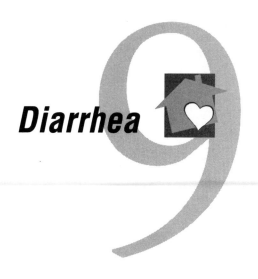

Diarrhea

1. UNDERSTANDING THE PROBLEM

Diarrhea is stools that are passed more often and in greater amounts than usual, and that are loose or liquid in consistency. With diarrhea, bowel movements usually feel urgent. Diarrhea causes the body to lose fluid, which leads to fatigue and to feeling "washed out" and which may also cause dehydration, a serious health problem. Controlling diarrhea is therefore very important for health as well as for comfort.

Chronic diarrhea is a common problem for persons with HIV/AIDS, and it frequently contributes to the HIV wasting syndrome (see the home care plan "HIV Wasting Syndrome" [Chapter 10]). The diarrhea may be caused by organisms (bacteria, fungi, viruses, and parasites) that infect the intestinal tract—usually because the immune system of the person with HIV/AIDS is too weakened to fight off the infection. Several medications used by persons with HIV/AIDS may also cause diarrhea. However, sometimes even after many tests have been done, no clear cause of the diarrhea is discovered.

> ➤ The information in this home care plan fits most situations, but yours may be different.
>
> ➤ If the doctor or nurse tells you to do something else, follow what he or she says.
>
> ➤ If you think there may be a medical emergency, see the section "When To Get Professional Help" on pp 98–99.

2. WHEN TO GET PROFESSIONAL HELP

Symptoms that indicate an emergency

Note: All of the following symptoms demand immediate attention. Severe diarrhea can result in a large amount of fluid loss. The problem is worse if

- The person you are caring for has already lost weight

- The diarrhea is accompanied by vomiting

- Additional fluid is being lost through perspiration

Dehydration then occurs quickly. Report severe diarrhea early so that medicines can be given to control it and so that fluids can be given.

Call the doctor, nurse, or "after hours" phone number *immediately* **if any of the following occurs:**

➤ **Severe diarrhea.**

With severe diarrhea, a great deal of fluid is being lost. Stools are very runny, and stomach cramps may occur. The severity of the problem depends on the person's weight and previous state of fluid balance. Severe diarrhea can quickly lead to dehydration. It is important to report this early so that medicines and fluids can be given to stop the diarrhea and correct the dehydration.

➤ **Blood in the diarrhea stool.**

Blood *in* the stool may signal bleeding in the lower intestine. Blood *around* a stool often indicates a rectal hemorrhoid, which is not an emergency. Sometimes it is hard to tell what caused the blood, so it is best to report it immediately.

➤ **Diarrhea accompanied by fever (temperature of more than 101 °F [38.3 °C]).**

Fever may be a sign of an intestinal infection. Dehydration may cause a slight fever, but in that case, the temperature is usually not higher than 101 °F.

➤ **Diarrhea accompanied by severe stomach pain.**

Severe stomach pain with diarrhea may indicate other problems, such as obstruction.

➤ **The person with diarrhea is lightheaded or dizzy when standing, or is too weak to stand up.**

These are signs of dehydration and low blood pressure. The body has lost too much fluid through diarrhea to work properly, and these fluids need to be replaced quickly.

➤ **Very little urine output during the past 24 hours.**

This is also a sign of dehydration.

➤ **Diarrhea accompanied by vomiting (occurs the same day as diarrhea).**

The medical staff needs to evaluate the causes of both the diarrhea and the vomiting. Also, the combination of the two can quickly lead to dehydration, so this needs to be reported immediately.

When you call, have the answers ready to the following questions:

1. What is the normal (usual) number of bowel movements per day for the person you are caring for?

2. How many bowel movements has he or she made during the past 24 hours?

3. Are the stools very liquid?

4. Is there any blood in the stool?

5. Do any other symptoms accompany the diarrhea?

   • Abdominal pain or cramps

   • Bloating or feeling full in the stomach or abdomen

   • Nausea

   • Vomiting

   • Redness, bleeding, cracking of the skin, or discharge from the rectal area

   • Fever

6. Has there been a change in diet recently? For example, has the person recently eaten raw fish or raw meat, or eaten at a picnic or restaurant?

7. How much liquid has the person drunk during the past 2 days (48 hours)? How much food has he or she eaten during the past 2 days?

8. What medicines has he or she taken during the past 2 to 3 days?

   • Any new medicines (prescribed or over-the-counter)

   • Antibiotics

   • Anti-diarrhea tablets or liquid

   • Other anti-infection medications

   • Any new "alternative" treatments

   • Any food supplements

9. Has the person you are caring for lost any weight? If so, how much over what period of time?

10. Does the person you are caring for have a history of other bowel problems such as diverticulitis, colitis, or irritable bowel syndrome?

11. Has the person you are caring for traveled recently?

12. Is anyone else at home also ill with diarrhea?

13. Does the person you are caring for become dizzy or lightheaded when standing?

14. How many hours per day does the person you are caring for need to spend in bed? How does this compare with what is usual for him or her?

Health care professionals need to know how much the person you are caring for is eating and drinking so that they can determine if the fluids being lost from the body are being replaced. Dehydration is a serious condition that can lead to dangerously low blood pressure and salt imbalance, and it needs to be treated as early as possible. Sometimes intravenous (IV) fluids need to be given to compensate for the fluid loss. These IV fluids may contain other substances that are being lost through the diarrhea, such as glucose, potassium, and sodium.

Here is an example of what you might say when calling for professional help:

"I am John Brown, Paul Smith's caregiver. Paul is a patient of Dr. Kroft. Paul has had diarrhea bowel movements six times today, and there is always blood mixed with the diarrhea stools."

3. WHAT YOU CAN DO TO HELP

> ### HERE ARE FOUR STEPS YOU CAN TAKE:
>
> Give medicines for diarrhea
>
> Replace lost fluids and nutrients
>
> Encourage the person you are caring for to avoid certain foods
>
> Increase comfort and protect the skin

Give medicines for diarrhea

➤ **Give anti-diarrhea medicine.**

These medicines slow down the working of the intestines. *Check with a health care professional before giving nonprescription medicines to stop diarrhea.* Certain anti-diarrhea medicines, even those sold over-the-counter, may actually make the problem worse. **Follow instructions on the label or prescription.** It is important to take anti-diarrhea medicines as directed and *to not take them more frequently than directed.*

Sometimes anti-diarrhea medicines do not work. Sometimes they work "too well" and cause constipation. These medicines may also cause sleepiness, even when only the recommended dose is given. If you encounter these problems, contact your doctor and discuss this with him or her.

Replace lost fluids and nutrients

Because important fluids and nutrients are lost with diarrhea, replacing them is crucial. Here are several ways of doing this:

➤ **Drink clear liquids.**

Clear liquids such as chicken broth, fruit juices, flat (noncarbonated) ginger ale, and Gatorade provide nourishment while allowing the bowel to rest. Clear liquids are also easier for the intestines to absorb into the bloodstream, and they quickly replace the fluids lost through diarrhea.

Diarrhea

➤ **Drink fluids between meals.**

Making sure to drink fluids *between* meals as well as during meals helps ensure that the body receives a steady amount of water and other nutrients. Usually, adults need 2 to 3 quarts (liters) of fluid each day if they have mild diarrhea, the same amount of fluid needed if they don't have diarrhea. They need more if they have severe diarrhea.

➤ **Eat low-fiber foods.**

Low-fiber foods do not "pull" water out of the body into the bowel the way high-fiber foods do. They are also easier to digest than high-fiber food. Examples of good low-fiber foods include bananas, rice, apple sauce, oatmeal, cranberries, strawberries, mashed potatoes, dry toast, crackers, eggs, fish, poultry, cottage cheese, and yogurt.

➤ **Eat small meals throughout the day instead of three large meals.**

Smaller meals are easier to digest. The person you are caring for will take in more fluid and food this way.

➤ **Eat high-potassium foods.**

Often, potassium is lost through diarrhea. This mineral is vital to the body and needs to be replaced. Examples of good high-potassium foods include apricot or peach nectar, bananas, and mashed or baked potatoes.

Encourage the person you are caring for to avoid certain foods

Some foods increase the action of the bowel or "pull" fluids out of body tissues into stool. Avoiding these foods may help reduce diarrhea:

➤ **Foods that produce gas: for example, beans, raw vegetables, raw fruits, broccoli, corn, cabbage, cauliflower, carbonated drinks, and chewing gum.**

➤ **Fatty foods, such as fatty meats and greasy fried food.**

Fats are difficult to digest. With diarrhea, the fats are pushed through without being digested, which adds to the diarrhea. If fat intolerance is a problem, you may want to substitute medium-chain triglycerides (MCT) oil for regular cooking oil in recipes and use nutritional supplements that contain MCT oil (Lipisorb, Osmolite, Nutren, and Peptamen).

➤ **Citrus fruits and juices, and alcohol.**

These drinks irritate the bowel and can cause diarrhea.

➤ **Avoid bran, nuts, seeds, and vegetables and fruits with skin.**

These foods are difficult to digest and can cause diarrhea.

➤ **Extremely hot food or hot drinks.**

Hot foods and liquids stimulate the bowel. Avoid these until the diarrhea is resolved.

➤ **Food and drinks that contain caffeine.**

Coffee, tea, some sodas (such as cola), and chocolate all contain caffeine. Caffeine makes the bowel work faster, and will make the diarrhea worse.

➤ **Milk and milk products (if they seem to make the diarrhea worse).**

Milk *may* make diarrhea worse for some people. It may also cause stomach cramps in some adults. Some nondairy foods, nutritional supplements, and medications may also contain lactose and should be avoided by people who are "lactose intolerant." Check labels.

Increase comfort and protect the skin

Diarrhea often causes discomfort. The intestinal cramping that can accompany diarrhea causes the lower abdomen to ache, and skin in the rectal area can become irritated and sore with each diarrhea stool. Here are some ways of dealing with abdominal cramping and skin soreness in the rectal area:

➤ **For abdominal cramping, use a hot water bottle or heating pad.**

Applying warmth to the abdomen can relieve pain and discomfort caused by cramping or tightness. Wrap the hot water bottle in a towel before applying it to the skin of the abdomen to avoid burning the skin or causing tenderness. Some people prefer to use an electric heating pad. Keep heating pads on a low, comfortable setting. *Do not put a heating pad on skin that has been radiated, burned, is broken, or has sores on it. Do not let the person you are caring for go to sleep with the heating pad on.*

➤ **For rectal skin soreness, cleanse the rectal area after each bowel movement.**

Cleansing helps prevent infection and further skin soreness. The person you are caring for should very gently cleanse the skin around the rectal area using warm water. This removes diarrhea stool, which can be very irritating. He or she should pat the skin dry, avoiding the friction of rubbing. A squirt bottle may also be tried for washing the skin; this sometimes removes stool more easily.

➤ **For rectal skin soreness, soak in warm water.**

Use the tub or a sitz bath to "soak away" soreness and to keep the rectal area clean. A sitz bath apparatus can be purchased at most pharmacies and medical equipment stores. Encourage the person with diarrhea to soak in warm water after each bowel movement or at least twice per day. If diarrhea is severe, however, and tends to come suddenly and without warning, tub soaking is not advisable.

➤ **For rectal skin soreness, apply soothing creams, ointments, or astringent pads such as Tucks to the rectal area.**

Creams prevent rectal skin from chapping in the same way that they prevent diaper rash or chapping on infant skin. Try Desitin, Nupercainal, A & D ointment, or Vaseline petroleum jelly. Astringent Tucks pads is another way of helping to dry the area and to soothe irritated skin. Also, because the creams or ointments serve as a protective layer to the skin, diarrhea will be less likely to cause a burning feeling.

➤ **Use adult diapers.**

Diarrhea that is constant or that comes on suddenly can be very embarrassing and also soils clothes and linens. One way to reduce these problems is to wear adult diapers. Adult diapers are available in stores or, if the person with HIV/AIDS is eligible for free supplies, can be obtained from the American Cancer Society.

➤ **For rectal soreness, wear underpants that are clean, dry, and loose.**

The rectal and genital areas can become very sore when diarrhea is a problem. Underwear should be loose and comfortable.

4. POSSIBLE OBSTACLES TO CAREGIVING

Here are some common attitudes and misconceptions that may prevent you from carrying out your plan:

"The person I'm caring for has had nothing to eat or drink for days, so this diarrhea can't last much longer."

Response: The body can keep removing fluid for much longer than you might think. The fluid is drawn from body tissues, and diarrhea can continue even if the person stops eating and drinking. It is very important to replace fluids that are lost.

"It's better to let the diarrhea 'run its course' because it is causing germs and bad organisms to leave the body."

Response: Diarrhea that is left to "run its course" may leave the person you are caring for dehydrated and extremely weakened. In a person whose immune system is working, diarrhea may sometimes resolve by itself. In persons with HIV/AIDS, however, diarrhea needs to be managed so that other problems, such as dehydration, do not arise.

Think of other obstacles

Identify additional roadblocks that could keep you from following the recommendations in this home care plan:

- Will the person I am caring for cooperate?

- Will other people help?

- How can I explain my needs to others?

- Do I have the time and energy to carry out this plan?

You need to develop plans for getting around these roadblocks. Use the four COPE ideas (Creativity, Optimism, Planning, and Expert information) in developing your plans. See pp 4–8 for a discussion of how to use the four COPE ideas in overcoming your obstacles.

5. CARRYING OUT AND ADJUSTING YOUR PLAN

Checking on results

Keep track of the frequency and severity of the diarrhea. Notice what causes diarrhea and what foods or fluids should be avoided. Also watch for progress in the comfort (for example, relief from rectal skin irritation) of the person you are caring for. Pay attention to which recommendations are working, and keep a "diary" of your progress.

What to do if your plan does not work

1. Review this chapter.

2. If you find that you've skipped something, try it now.

3. If you find that you've done all that you can, call the doctor for further guidance.

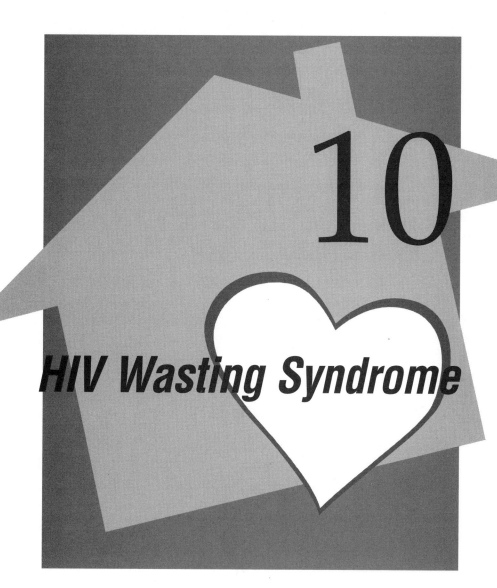

10

HIV Wasting Syndrome

Overview of the Home Care Plan for
HIV Wasting Syndrome

 1. UNDERSTANDING THE PROBLEM

> Recognizing HIV wasting syndrome
>
> Contributing factors
>
> Your goals

 2. WHEN TO GET PROFESSIONAL HELP

> Symptoms that indicate the need for professional help
>
> Information to have ready when you call
>
> What to say when you call

 3. WHAT YOU CAN DO TO HELP

> Encourage gaining weight and improving nutrition
>
> Encourage conserving energy and help to increase activity
>
> Provide for the safety of the person you are caring for

 4. POSSIBLE OBSTACLES

5. CARRYING OUT AND ADJUSTING YOUR PLAN

> Carrying out your plan
>
> Checking on results
>
> What to do if your plan does not work

Topics that have an arrow (➤) in front of them are actions you can take or symptoms you can look for.

HIV Wasting Syndrome

1. UNDERSTANDING THE PROBLEM

Weight loss and weakness are common among persons with HIV/AIDS. However, weight loss and weakness, accompanied by other symptoms, may be a sign of the AIDS-related condition known as HIV wasting syndrome. Malnutrition is the major cause of the HIV wasting syndrome. A person who has this syndrome develops a worn, wasted appearance similar to that of a starving person. The malnutrition is usually the result of eating problems such as (1) decreased eating due to fatigue; (2) loss of appetite; (3) infection in the mouth or gastrointestinal tract; (4) poor absorption of fatty foods; and (4) poor absorption of foods, in general, because of diarrhea. HIV wasting syndrome may be worsened by other illnesses, as well as by the side effects of medications used to treat HIV/AIDS. This home care plan focuses on HIV wasting syndrome and not on other causes of weight loss, such as tumors, infections, or loss of appetite.

> ➤ The information in this home care plan fits most situations, but yours may be different.
>
> ➤ If the doctor or nurse tells you to do something else, follow what he or she says.
>
> ➤ If you think there may be a medical emergency, see the section "When To Get Professional Help" on pp 110–111.

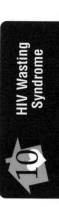

HIV Wasting Syndrome

Wasting cannot be "cured" simply by food or good nutrition. It is important not to focus on making the person you are caring for eat. He or she may feel defeated, or tension may increase unnecessarily. Some home caregivers find themselves pushing food and neglecting many other important things, such as spending relaxed time with the person with HIV/AIDS.

YOUR GOALS

Know when to call for professional help

Encourage gaining weight and improving nutrition

Encourage conserving energy and help to increase activity

Provide for the safety of the person you are caring for

WHEN TO GET PROFESSIONAL HELP

Each symptom of HIV wasting syndrome is serious by itself. If several problems are occurring at the same time, they can reduce energy, enthusiasm, and the will to face a new day.

Call the doctor or nurse if any of the following occurs:

➤ **Weight loss of greater than 10% of total body weight or 10 to 15 pounds over a 6- to 8-week period.**

A weight loss of more than 10% of a person's total body weight is generally 10 to 15 pounds. Such a weight loss is characteristic of HIV wasting syndrome (unless it is brought on by dieting). Weight loss of greater than 10% of total body weight in less than 6 to 8 weeks indicates that more is occurring than the normal wasting syndrome. Diagnosing its cause and treating it are very important.

➤ **Marked weakness.**

Weakness that prevents a person from caring for himself or herself (that is, everyday self care, such as toileting, dressing, or washing the face and hands) and from activity such as visiting with others or eating is another characteristic of HIV wasting syndrome. The weakness is also *chronic* and usually accompanies dramatic weight loss. These feelings of fatigue do not necessarily improve with rest. (See the home care plan "Fatigue" [Chapter 12].)

➤ **Fevers of 99 to 101 °F for 30 days or longer.**

Such fevers are caused by HIV or by active infection in the lungs, brain, gastrointestinal tract, or elsewhere. Fevers speed up the body's metabolism (ability to burn calories) and lead to more weight loss or wasting. (See the home care plan "Fever" [Chapter 5].)

➤ **Chronic diarrhea.**

See the home care plan "Diarrhea" (Chapter 9).

When you call, have the answers to the following questions ready:

1. Is the person you are caring for avoiding eating? If so, what do you believe is the cause? (For example, diarrhea, mouth or throat problems, lack of energy, shortness of breath, forgetfulness, cramping and abdominal pain after eating, or loss of appetite due to fever or nausea and/or vomiting.)

2. During the past 24 hours, how much food has the person you are caring for eaten and how much fluid has he or she drunk? (Make a list of the specific foods and drinks, and report these to the health care professional.)

3. Has the person you are caring for had diarrhea during the past 24 hours? If so, how many bowel movements has he or she had during this period? What is the amount and color of the stools? Is there blood present, or do the stools have a bad odor?

4. Has the person you are caring for been losing weight? How much weight has he or she lost during the past 6 to 8 weeks?

5. How often does the person you are caring for have fevers? How high do they get? How are you treating the fevers?

6. Are the fevers accompanied by other problems such as a rash, cough, headache, abdominal pain, or eye problems?

7. Is the person you are caring for fatigued and weak? Does he or she refuse to get out of bed? How many hours does he or she spend in bed each day?

8. Has the person you are caring for experienced a fall (for example, in the home) because of weakness? When walking, does he or she need to hold onto things to prevent falling?

9. Is the person you are caring for very thin? (Give his or her height and weight.)

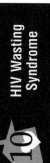

10. Does he or she shy away from others? Is he or she discouraged because of not having success in gaining weight or strength?

11. Is the person you are caring for on a special diet or using an "alternative therapy" that involves the gastrointestinal tract?

Here is an example of what you might say when calling for professional help:

"I am May Green, Paul Green's caregiver. Paul is a patient of Dr. Smith. Paul is losing weight rapidly and has been growing very weak and thin. He has lost 15 pounds over the past 5 weeks. He looks so frail, and his clothes just hang on him. He has also been having a great deal of diarrhea."

3. WHAT YOU CAN DO TO HELP

HERE ARE THREE STEPS YOU CAN TAKE:

Encourage gaining weight and improving nutrition

Encourage conserving energy and help to increase activity

Provide for the safety of the person you are caring for

Encourage gaining weight and improving nutrition

Many factors, such as loss of appetite, nausea, and mouth and throat infection, are related to weight loss and poor nutrition. The home care plans "Problems with Appetite" (Chapter 6), "Nausea and Vomiting" (Chapter 8), and "Problems with the Mouth" (Chapter 7) discuss these subjects in detail and provide many suggestions for improving nutrition and weight gain.

➤ **Improve appetite and promote weight gain.**

You can help improve the appetite of the person you are caring for by making mealtime more pleasant, by making foods more appealing, and by preventing an early sense of "fullness." The home care plan "Problems with Appetite" (Chapter 6) provides these and other suggestions for improving the appetite, as well as gives recommendations on how to make foods more nutritious and calorie-rich.

> ### Prevent and treat nausea and vomiting.

Nausea and vomiting may contribute to poor appetite and weight loss. The home care plan "Nausea and Vomiting" (Chapter 8) offers suggestions on how to decrease these symptoms.

> ### Treat mouth sores and infections early.

Viral and fungal infections can create problems not only in the mouth but also in the gastrointestinal tract. Consult the home care plan "Problems with the Mouth" for a discussion on how to treat the mouth and throat problems that interfere with eating.

Encourage conserving energy and help to increase activity

People with HIV wasting syndrome have a low energy level and are usually tired after minimal exertion. Here are several ways you can help the person you are caring for to conserve energy.

> ### Balance periods of activity and rest.

This will prevent the person you are caring for from becoming excessively fatigued. The home care plan "Fatigue" (Chapter 12) includes suggestions on how to balance periods of activity with periods of rest.

> ### Encourage the person you are caring for to remain as active as possible to avoid further physical or emotional setbacks.

When the person with HIV/AIDS feels "slowed down" and weak, remaining active becomes more difficult. He or she may want to move less, stay in bed more, and keep activities to a bare minimum. This can create physical problems such as muscle weakness, skin breakdown (bed sores), and an increased chance of getting pneumonia. This can also lead to emotional problems such as depression and feelings of worthlessness. Therefore, even when the person is feeling tired, he or she should try to keep as active as possible.

> ### Plan activities for periods of the day when the energy level is the highest.

Determine what times of the day the person you are caring for is feeling best, and then encourage personal hygiene and grooming, social activities, and activities that are pleasant or fun (for example, taking a walk) for those times of the day. Having a fixed, daily routine, with rest periods when needed, will produce the best results. A daily routine also allows the person to match his or

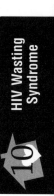

her energy level with a necessary activity level—and this is satisfying for both caregiver and patient.

> ### Avoid the "doing for" syndrome.

Caregivers often feel guilty if they refuse to do something for the person they are caring for. They may find themselves doing more and more, and the person they are helping doing less and less. This pattern will only add to the weakness and inactivity of the person you are caring for. Learn to say a kind "no." Try to adopt a "do for yourself" policy, whenever possible.

Provide for the safety of the person you are caring for

Safety is a big concern when the person with HIV/AIDS becomes weakened. A person who is weakened is more prone to falls, which may, in turn, may lead to a fear of "future" falls, causing him or her to avoid activity. Here are some ways of ensuring safety and of preventing unnecessary fears:

> ### Encourage the use of assist devices.

At some point, the person you are caring for may need to use a walker, wheelchair, commode, or handrails. He or she may see these devices as representing a loss of independence and as signs that he or she has grown much sicker, and may therefore refuse to use any such equipment. You should help him or her see assist devices as aids to staying independent, rather than as signs of dependency.

> ### Keep the home hazard-free.

When the AIDS virus affects nerves that control muscle movements, the way the person moves will change. You may see the person you are caring for stagger when walking, stumble, or fall. Loose rugs are very easy to slip on and should be removed from linoleum and wooden floor surfaces. To prevent tripping, you should also remove obstacles that clutter or block walking areas inside the home, such as toys and decorative objects. Try to keep the home as uncluttered as possible. Also, when taking a walk outside the home with him or her, make sure that the path you take is clear.

> ### Equip the bathroom with safety devices.

Most falls occur in the bathroom. Install handrails in the shower or tub and around the toilet. Shower chairs make bathing or showering much safer. The larger the chair or bench, the more steady it will be. Nonslip appliqués, placed on the bottom of the tub, make getting in and out much safer.

➤ **Raise beds, toilet seats, chairs, and couches for easier transfers.**

When the height of a regular bed is too low, getting in and out of it can be difficult. If this is the case, raise the bed on wooden blocks to make moving in or out safer and easier. Toilets, too, are often too low for the person who is feeling weak and unsteady. Raised toilet seats, which are commonly used by persons who have arthritis or who have had hip surgery, elevate the toilet seat 4 to 6 inches. These toilet seats are usually made of sturdy plastic and are relatively inexpensive. Wooden blocks or platforms can be placed under easychairs or couches, making it easier to sit down and to get up again.

➤ **Place sliding boards between seats for difficult transfers.**

When the person you are caring for is too weak to transfer from a bed to a wheelchair, or from a chair to a commode, sliding boards are helpful. These are short pieces of wood that stretch between the two surfaces. He or she does not have to stand to do the transfer but instead slides or eases the body across the board to the new site. Sliding boards are helpful not only when the person you are caring for is feeling weak but also when no one is available to help him or her move and when the caregiver is physically unable to lift or help the person to switch places.

➤ **Obtain medical equipment for use in the home.**

Surgical supply stores or companies that manufacture durable medical equipment have catalogs of materials needed for the home, such as wheelchairs, commodes, shower handrails, or bath chairs. Ask to see these catalogs so that you can consider what is needed for your home and how much it costs. Sometimes certain service groups or organizations such as the VFW, the American Cancer Society, and the Lions Club have "used" equipment to donate or lend. They may also sponsor fund-raising campaigns to buy equipment that is needed. Call the Center for Disease Control's National AIDS Hotline at 1-800-342-AIDS, or call your local AIDS Service Organization (ASO) to find out what help is available. You might also speak with a health care professional or social worker about obtaining equipment to use at home.

➤ **Assist the person you are caring for with his or her daily activities.**

Numbness, weakness, tingling, and tremors in the hands can interfere with the person's ability to prepare a meal, feed himself or herself, shave, dress, and bathe. Provide assistance, when needed, without taking away from the person's sense of independence. Consult the nurse, social worker, or occupational therapist about purchasing or borrowing devices that help with cooking, eating, or bathing. Also, clothing can be adjusted to allow for self-care. For example, Velcro strips can replace buttons, or tops with button-down fronts can be substituted for pullover tops.

➤ **Monitor the use of pain medicines and medicines that make the mood more stable.**

If the memory of the person you are caring for has been affected, he or she may forget to take medicines in the proper quantity and at the correct time. Setting up medications beforehand, posting reminders around the home, or using an alarm clock as a reminder may help. If necessary, you should control the medication supply, dispensing small amounts of medicine for certain hours of the day. (See the home care plan "Opportunistic Infections" [Chapter 4], pp 45–46, for more suggestions on how to supervise the use of medications.)

➤ **Consider using Life Line or other emergency response systems.**

Life Line is a device that is worn around the neck or placed near the person, allowing the wearer to press a button to summon help when needed. As many as three persons can usually be alerted. The electronic device sends a signal to a phone in a central office, which, in turn, contacts the people or agencies you designate.

4. POSSIBLE OBSTACLES TO CAREGIVING

Here are some common attitudes and misconceptions that may prevent you from carrying out your plan:

"I'm glad that I have lost weight. I was overweight before."

Response: Weight loss for the person with HIV wasting syndrome can be dramatic. Most persons do not realize this until they have lost as much as 20 pounds and are continuing to lose weight. Weight loss needs to be combated early, even if the person feels that he or she looks "better" after losing weight. Notify the doctor about the weight loss, and review this chapter for suggestions on how to regain the weight that has been lost.

"Wheelchairs, walkers, and canes are for old people. I don't need them yet."

Response: Help the person you are caring for to understand that these devices can help him or her be safe, active, and independent. A physical therapist can give instructions on how to use them. If the person you are caring for is reluctant to have others see him or her use assist devices, put them away during visits. You can bring them back when the visitors are gone.

Think of other obstacles

Identify additional roadblocks that could keep you from following the recommendations of this home care plan:

- Will the person I am caring for cooperate?
- Will other people help?
- How can I explain my needs to others?
- Do I have the time and energy to carry out this plan?

You need to develop plans for getting around these roadblocks. Use the four COPE ideas (Creativity, Optimism, Planning, and Expert information) in developing your plans. See pp 4–8 for a discussion of how to use the four COPE ideas.

5. CARRYING OUT AND ADJUSTING YOUR PLAN

Carrying out your plan

Sometimes the symptoms of HIV wasting syndrome may be brought to your attention simply by your *noticing* them, not because the person you are caring for discusses them with you. He or she may be experiencing weakness, weight loss, decreased mobility, and less independence but may be unwilling to talk about it. In this case, it is up to *you* to start the conversation and to be honest. Assure him or her that many steps can be taken to solve these problems. Both you and the person you are caring for must be open and honest with each other to manage these problems effectively. Remember that ignoring symptoms will only result in larger problems that are harder to solve. Act early, using the suggestions in this plan.

Checking on results

Keep track of the problems that occur. Pay attention to which recommendations are working, and keep a "diary" of your progress.

What to do if your plan does not work

1. Review this chapter.

2. If you find that you've skipped something, try it now.

3. If you find that you've done all you can, call the doctor for further guidance.

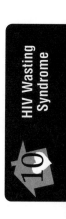

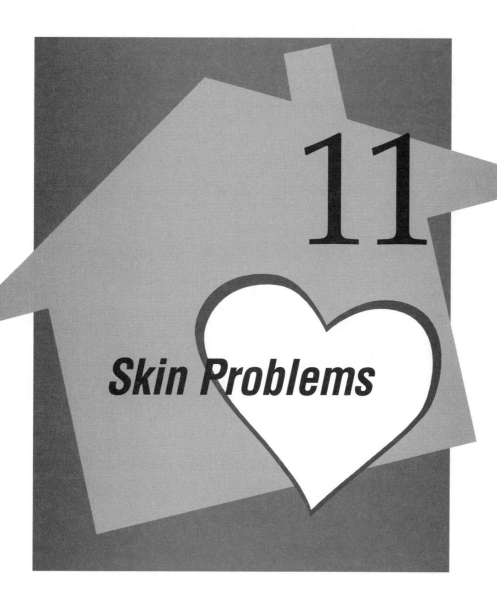

11

Skin Problems

Overview of the Home Care Plan for
Skin Problems

1. UNDERSTANDING THE PROBLEM

> Types of skin problems associated with HIV/AIDS
>
> Causes of skin problems
>
> Your goals

2. WHEN TO GET PROFESSIONAL HELP

> Symptoms that indicate the need for professional help
>
> Information to have ready when you call
>
> What to say when you call

3. WHAT YOU CAN DO TO HELP

> Care for the skin during and after radiation therapy
>
> Relieve and prevent itching and dryness
>
> Treat skin rashes and eruptions
>
> Prevent skin breakdown
>
> Keep skin problems from becoming worse

4. POSSIBLE OBSTACLES TO CAREGIVING

5. CARRYING OUT AND ADJUSTING YOUR PLAN

> Checking on results
>
> What to do if your plan does not work

**Topics that have an arrow (➤) in front
of them are actions you can take or
symptoms you can look for.**

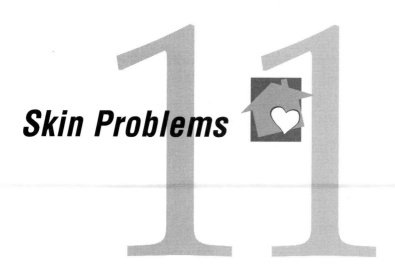

Skin Problems

1. Understanding the Problem

The person with HIV/AIDS may experience any of several skin problems. These may look unpleasant and may feel uncomfortable, painful, or irritating. They may also indicate a more serious problem.

Some skin problems, such as redness, irritation, rashes, itching, peeling, and changes in skin color, may be side effects of medications used to treat HIV/AIDS. For example, the radiation therapy used to treat Kaposi's sarcoma (an abnormal skin growth related to HIV/AIDS) can darken the skin.

Another cause of skin problems is infection. The fungus *Candida albicans*, which causes the mouth infection called *thrush*, can also result in rashes that occur around the groin, penis, vagina, and rectal area and which itch and spread easily. One type of herpes virus may cause

> ➤ The information in this home care plan fits most situations, but yours may be different.
>
> ➤ If the doctor or nurse tells you to do something else, follow what he or she says.
>
> ➤ If you think there may be a medical emergency, see the section "When To Get Professional Help" on pp 122–123.

"fever blisters" that form on the lips. Another type of herpes virus (herpes zoster) is responsible for a very painful rash known as "shingles."

Kaposi's sarcoma is a type of growth that a person with HIV/AIDS may acquire. These "tumors" usually appear on the skin but can also affect some of the organs within the body.

> ## YOUR GOALS
>
> Know when to call for professional help
>
> Care for the skin during and after radiation therapy
>
> Relieve and prevent itching and dryness
>
> Treat skin rashes and eruptions
>
> Prevent skin breakdown
>
> Keep skin problems from becoming worse

WHEN TO GET PROFESSIONAL HELP

Call the doctor or nurse if any of the following occurs:

➤ **Skin rashes are spreading or draining or are made up of small blisters.**

These rashes may point to a drug reaction or to an infection that needs to be treated. If ignored for too long, problematic rashes will cause more severe symptoms, such as infection or skin breakdown.

➤ **A new raised purple flat area appears on various parts of the body.**

Purple skin spots may be Kaposi's sarcoma. These are growths or nodules that are blue to purple in color, appearing on the legs, trunk, arms, head, or neck.

➤ **A new rash or hives.**

New rashes or hives (especially when blisters appear on the head, neck, or upper chest area) may signal an allergic reaction to a medicine. In this case, the medicine may need to be changed or its dosage decreased.

➤ **Severe itching that lasts for more than 1 day.**

Itching is a bothersome side effect that may be caused by a reaction to medication, or infection. The doctor may prescribe medication to relieve the itching. A quick relief of the itching is always desirable.

➤ **Pressure sores.**

Persons with HIV/AIDS who have lost a great deal of weight and who are less active and more weak may develop pressure sores. Pressure sores (also known as *bed sores*) are usually caused by lying in bed in the same position for several hours at a time. At first the bedsore will appear pink, then red, and finally, will open up as a deep, draining sore. All pressure sores should be reported early so that treatment can begin without delay.

When you call, have the answers ready to the following questions:

1. If the person you are caring for has a rash, where on the body is it located? Does the rash itch or hurt? What does it look like?

2. When did the skin problem start?

3. What do you think caused it?

4. How serious, uncomfortable, or embarrassing is the skin problem?

5. What medicines are he or she taking? Have any of these been started just recently?

6. What have you done thus far to treat the skin problem and has this improved the skin problem at all?

7. Does he or she have a fever?

8. Has he or she been exposed to ultraviolet light or sunlight recently?

9. Has he or she had any recent change in diet?

10. Have he or she changed soaps, detergents, creams, or perfumes lately?

11. Is he or she using a new "alternative therapy?"

The answers to these questions will help the health care professional pinpoint not only the duration and severity of the problem but also its origin.

Here is an example of what you might say when calling for professional help:

"This is Fred Johnson, Steve Green's caregiver. Steve is patient of Dr. Brown. Steve has a rash on his chest and abdomen that itches severely. Steve started a new drug, Bactrim, last week. What should I do?"

3. WHAT YOU CAN DO TO HELP

> **HERE ARE FIVE STEPS YOU CAN TAKE:**
>
> Care for the skin during and after radiation therapy
>
> Relieve and prevent itching and dryness
>
> Treat skin rashes and eruptions
>
> Prevent skin breakdown
>
> Keep skin problems from becoming worse

Care for the skin during and after radiation therapy

Some persons with HIV/AIDS may acquire AIDS-related growths or cancer. The most common are Kaposi's sarcoma and non-Hodgkin's lymphoma. Radiation therapy is sometimes the treatment of choice for these conditions. In this case, good skin care is necessary. Ask the oncologist or radiation therapist for specific instructions in the care of radiated skin.

Here are some ways to care for the skin after radiation therapy:

➤ **On areas of the skin that have received radiation treatments, avoid using the following:**

- Scented or medicated lotions

- Rubbing alcohol

- Creams

- Body oils

- Talcum powder or cornstarch

- Perfumes

- Antiperspirants

These irritate the skin, and many leave a coating that actually interferes with radiation therapy or healing. A special cream may be prescribed by the radiation therapist, who will explain how to use it.

➤ **Report wet or damp skin areas to radiation clinic staff.**

The radiation clinic staff will give you suggestions on how to treat wet or damp skin areas if they are near areas that have been treated by radiation. Wet or moist areas are more likely to appear in skin folds, under the arms, and in the groin.

➤ **Avoid the use of ice packs.**

Ice irritates the skin. It also constricts the blood vessels, which may inhibit healing.

➤ **Avoid direct sunlight.**

The ultraviolet rays of the sun can burn radiation-treated skin easily because the skin layer is very tender during and after radiation therapy. The person you are caring for should avoid direct sun exposure for at least 1 year after radiation treatments.

➤ **Wear loose-fitting clothing.**

Tight-fitting clothing causes redness and irritation, whereas loose-fitting clothing lets the skin breathe and does not restrict its flexibility.

Relieve and prevent itching and dryness

Here are some ways to relieve and prevent itching and dryness:

➤ **Bathe with cool water, using gentle soap.**

Hot water and harsh soaps can dry and damage skin tissue very easily. Try an oatmeal soap or one that contains oil (soap with any special oil will be labeled as such). Alpha Keri, which eliminates the need for soap while it softens the skin, may be added to bath water.

➤ **Limit bathing to a few times per week.**

Although many people are accustomed to bathing daily, frequent baths may dry out the skin. Wash face, hands, and personal areas every day, but full baths should be limited to a few times each week. Sponge baths are another means of decreasing the amount of warm water on the skin.

➤ **Add baking soda, mineral oil, or baby oil to bath water.**

Baking soda soothes sensitive skin and decreases itching. Mineral oil or baby oil will soak in and prevent the water from drying out the skin. Also, after a bath or shower, mineral oil should be applied to the skin before it is patted dry, leaving the skin very moist. The person you are caring for should wear sweatpants and a long-sleeved shirt to help retain moisture on the skin for 1 hour after bathing. Wet or oily clothing should be removed after 1 hour.

> **Avoid scrubbing the skin.**

Scrubbing pulls on delicate skin tissue and removes important moisture.

> **Rinse the skin thoroughly and pat it dry.**

Removing soap and perspiration from the skin by rinsing it well will relieve some of the itching. Patting the skin dry can prevent further irritation of affected areas.

> **Apply cool, moist compresses to itching skin.**

Cool soaks are soothing and relieve itching at least for a short time. Use washcloths or soft dish towels soaked in cool water.

> **Change bed sheets often.**

Dry skin tends to "flake off" and gather on bed sheets, which, in turn, can cause more itchiness. Unclean sheets also acquire a buildup of bacteria. Changing the sheets frequently will help eliminate these problems. Fresh sheets also give a sense of comfort.

> **Avoid harsh laundry detergents.**

Harsh detergents remain on clothes, causing itching and irritation. Try rewashing clothing without adding any soap to the second cycle to rinse off detergents. Using fragrance-free laundry soap and fabric softener may help, too.

> **Keep the room temperature cool, and avoid extreme heat or cold.**

Try to keep the room temperature as comfortable as possible. When a person perspires, itching increases.

> **Drink 2 to 3 quarts of fluids every day, unless otherwise instructed.**

Drinking plenty of fluids reduces the risk of dehydration and restores needed moisture to skin tissue.

> **Use an electric razor.**

Electric razors are less likely to scrape off layers of skin.

Treat skin rashes and eruptions

Here are ways of treating rashes and eruptions (blisters or pimples):

> **Keep the skin clean and dry.**

Skin rashes caused by infections become more uncomfortable and tend to spread if the skin is not kept clean and dry. Do not apply antiperspirants or deodorants to the rash area. Cleanse the skin with mild soap and warm water. Scented soaps or deodorant soaps tend to be harsh on the skin, often inflaming it even more. Clear soaps or oatmeal soaps are milder.

➤ **Wash infected areas separately.**

Have a separate washcloth for washing areas that have rashes, infections, or skin eruptions. This helps limit the spread of infection to other areas.

➤ **Apply prescribed medication on affected areas.**

The prescribed medication may be medicated ointments, lotions, creams, or powders. Affected skin areas should be cleaned and dried before every new application.

➤ **Treat *everyone* in the household if parasitic insects are the cause of the rashes or eruptions.**

If the doctor thinks that the rash is caused by parasitic insects such as fleas, lice, or mites, it is important to treat *everyone* who lives in the same household as the person you are caring for. Wash all clothes and bed linens in hot water on the *same day*.

➤ **Treat folliculitis as directed by a health care professional.**

Although some people who have folliculitis (an inflammation of the hair follicles) use solutions containing alcohol to dry up erupted areas, alcohol can make the skin too dry and itchy. The best treatment for this problem is good skin cleansing and therapies suggested by a nurse or physician.

➤ **Use medicated shampoos for scaly lesions on the hair line.**

Some persons with HIV/AIDS may have seborrheic dermatitis, an inflammatory skin disease in which yellowish crusting and scaling occurs at the hairline, eyebrows, ear region, and around the nose. Shampooing with a medicated shampoo (such as a dandruff shampoo) is helpful.

Prevent skin breakdown

Persons with HIV/AIDS often experience weight loss, weakness, and a decreased level of activity. Skin problems such as bedsores and skin breakdown can result from sitting or lying in bed all day. Here are some steps you can take to prevent these skin problems:

➤ **Change positions every 2 hours.**

If the person you are caring for remains in bed for most of the day, have him or her change position every 2 hours to prevent skin soreness and breakdown.

> **Use pressure-relieving devices.**

Acquire pressure-relieving devices for bed and chairs, such as foam pads or mattresses, air mattresses or cushions (pad must be at least 4 inches thick), and the more sophisticated "alternating pressure devices." These help to keep pressure off bony areas of the body.

> **Keep linens clean, smooth, and dry.**

Keep linens dry, clean, and without wrinkles. This will help to protect the skin. This is especially important when the person you are caring for is incontinent.

> **Use sheepskin pads under the hips and on heels and elbows, as needed.**

These pads, when used under the hips and on heels and elbows, prevent friction and rubbing of delicate skin on the bed sheets.

> **Massage reddened areas caused by pressure.**

Massaging reddened areas with body lotions or creams (during very short massages—i.e., *less than 1 minute*) promotes circulation to the skin and can keep these areas from developing into pressure sores. (However, do not use lotion during the *longer* massage, because it softens the skin too much and can make the skin break down.)

> **Serve high-protein foods.**

Good nutrition is important in preventing skin breakdown, as well as in promoting skin healing.

> **Use an easy-chair or reclining chair during the day.**

Padded chairs that recline are comfortable, permit a shifting of body weight, and keep the legs elevated to prevent swelling. Sitting up is a must.

Keep skin problems from becoming worse

Here are some ways to keep existing skin problems from becoming worse:

> **Report a worsening skin condition.**

It is important to report (during office hours) any condition of the skin that looks or feels worse. Give the doctor or nurse a clear description of how the skin looks. Describe how it has changed over the last few days and what you have done to treat the problem.

➤ **Discontinue remedies if the problem gets worse.**

Use the remedies and skin care techniques that the doctor or nurse has suggested. If you are following his or her recommendations and the skin problem gets worse, discontinue the treatment and contact them. If the condition improves, continue the treatment and the other things you are doing to treat skin problems on your own.

➤ **Discourage the person you are caring for from scratching the skin.**

Scratching irritated skin usually causes it to become raw and more uncomfortable. Discourage this habit through gentle reminders to the person you are caring for. Sometimes wearing cotton gloves is helpful, especially at night, to prevent scratching. Also, applying some pressure to the itchy area with a warm hand may help.

POSSIBLE OBSTACLES TO CAREGIVING

Here are some common attitudes and misconceptions that may prevent you from carrying out your plan:

"It's only the skin, so it's not a 'real' problem."

Response: Seemingly trivial skin problems may lead to infection and other serious problems, and therefore need to be treated early. Watch for changes in the skin and do not wait until an infection or severe discomfort occurs.

"No one seems to know what to do about this itching. I guess I'll just have to live with it."

Response: Although itching is a very difficult problem to get rid of, you should not "give up." Try a combination of the strategies in this home care plan to relieve constant itching. Keep experimenting.

Think of other obstacles

Identify additional roadblocks that could keep you from following the recommendations in this home care plan:

• Will the person I am caring for cooperate?

• Will other people help?

• How can I explain my needs to others?

• Do I have the time and energy to carry out this plan?

You need to develop plans for getting around these roadblocks. Use the four COPE ideas (Creativity, Optimism, Planning, and Expert information) in developing your plans. See pp 4–8 for a discussion on how to use the four COPE ideas.

5. CARRYING OUT AND ADJUSTING YOUR PLAN

Checking on results

Keep track of skin problems, while watching for changes or signs that the skin conditions may be becoming worse. Pay attention to which recommendations are working, and keep a "diary" of your progress.

What to do if your plan does not work

1. Review this chapter.

2. If you find that you've skipped something, try it now.

3. If you find that you've done all that you can, call the doctor for further guidance.

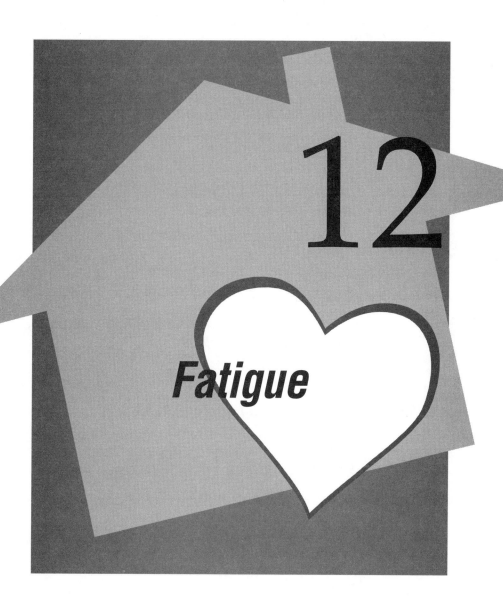

12

Fatigue

Overview of the Home Care Plan for
Fatigue

 1. UNDERSTANDING THE PROBLEM

      Causes of fatigue in persons with HIV/AIDS

      Your goals

 2. WHEN TO GET PROFESSIONAL HELP

      Symptoms that indicate an emergency

      Symptoms that do not indicate an emergency but should be reported

      Information to have ready when you call

      What to say when you call

 3. WHAT YOU CAN DO TO HELP

      Plan rest, activity, and nutrition

      Promote rest and sleep

 4. POSSIBLE OBSTACLES TO CAREGIVING

5. CARRYING OUT AND ADJUSTING YOUR PLAN

      Checking on results

      What to do if your plan does not work

Topics that have an arrow (➤) in front of them are actions you can take or symptoms you can look for.

Fatigue

 1. ## UNDERSTANDING THE PROBLEM

Persons with HIV/AIDS often feel "worn out" and tired. Fatigue usually increases as the disease progresses. HIV has a "wearing" and "wasting" effect on many parts of the body, leading to low energy and fatigue. Persons with HIV/AIDS are also more prone to acquire infections because of the damage the virus causes to the immune system, the body's protective mechanism. Infections, the symptoms they cause, and the aggressive treatment that they require take their toll, leaving the person with HIV/AIDS with decreased resistance and strength.

> ➤ The information in this home care plan fits most situations, but yours may be different.
>
> ➤ If the health care professional tells you to do something else, follow what he or she says.
>
> ➤ If you think there may be a medical emergency, see the section "When To Get Professional Help" on pp 134–135.

Many of the medicines used to treat HIV/AIDS may also produce fatigue. Emotional stress caused by the illness can also contribute to tiredness in persons with HIV/AIDS.

Your GOALS

Know when to get professional help

Plan rest, activity, and nutrition

Promote rest and sleep

2. WHEN TO GET PROFESSIONAL HELP

Although fatigue itself is not an emergency, some of the symptoms that accompany fatigue are serious.

Symptoms that indicate an emergency

Call the doctor, nurse, or "after hours" phone number *immediately* if any of the following conditions accompany fatigue:

➤ **Severe or frequent dizziness.**

Although occasional dizziness is common even in healthy persons, severe or frequent dizziness should be reported to a health care professional immediately. *Severe* dizziness lasts about 3 to 4 minutes and makes the person feel a spinning sensation. *Frequent* dizziness may be less severe and may not last as long, but the dizziness happens almost every time the person changes positions, such as going from sitting to standing.

➤ **Injury, bleeding, mental confusion, or a "black out" caused by a fall.**

Report all bad falls and what caused the fall so that the doctor can determine whether bones are broken or if the head has received a serious blow. The doctor can then decide what follow-up is needed.

➤ **Inability to wake up.**

Call 911 or the medical care clinic *immediately* if you cannot awaken the person you are caring for. He or she will probably need to be taken to a medical facility for tests to determine the cause of this problem.

➤ **Breathlessness.**

Breathlessness, or "feeling out of breath," usually occurs because the body is not getting the right amount of oxygen. This can be caused by a respiratory problem or a low level of red blood cells.

> ### Inability to perform daily activities.

A sudden change in the ability to perform daily activities, such as dressing or eating, is a reason to call for help immediately.

Symptoms that do not indicate an emergency but should be reported during regular office or clinic hours

> ### Ringing in the ears.

Ringing in the ears may be caused by a reaction to medication, a change in blood flow to the brain, or other physical changes. Medical tests are usually required to determine its cause.

> ### Pounding in the head.

Pounding in the head also signals a problem with blood flow or blood pressure. Medical tests are usually required to determine its cause.

> ### Excessive bed rest.

If the person you are caring for stays in bed for days, this may be a sign of severe depression, particularly if it continues for several days without other symptoms. Severe depression needs to be reported to a health care professional. (For a more detailed discussion, see the home care plan "Coping with Depression" [Chapter 17].)

> ### Severe headaches.

Severe headaches can cause fatigue and should be reported.

When you call, have the answers ready to the following questions:

1. Does the person you are caring for seem to be thinking more unclearly than before the symptoms occurred?

2. Has he or she experienced any confusion or has confusion grown worse since the fatigue increased?

3. Is he or she feeling depressed?

4. Has he or she started any new medicine (prescribed or over-the-counter), such as pain medicine or sleep medicine?

5. Has he or she started any new "alternative therapies"?

Here is an example of what you might say when calling for professional help:

"I am Paul Clark, Harry Smith's caregiver. Harry is Dr. Kline's patient. Harry has been feeling dizzy and weak every time he gets up and tries to walk around the house. This started 2 days ago."

3. WHAT YOU CAN DO TO HELP

> **HERE ARE TWO STEPS YOU CAN TAKE:**
>
> Plan rest, activity, and nutrition
>
> Promote rest and sleep

Plan rest, activity, and nutrition

➤ **Plan the day so that activities occur when the person you are caring for feels most refreshed and awake.**

Plan activities during the time of day or evening when the person feels best. Allow time for rest between activities.

➤ **Encourage rest before activities.**

Encourage rest *before* activities you know will be tiring. This will not only help ensure that he or she does not become "tired out" but will also make the activities more enjoyable.

➤ **Encourage conserving energy.**

The person you are caring for can conserve energy by engaging in activities for short periods only. Also, encourage him or her to do only those things that give him or her enjoyment, or that are absolutely necessary.

➤ **Get help with child care.**

If the person you are caring for has children, do what you can to limit the work involved with the children and increase the quality time he or she spends with them.

➤ **Encourage moving slowly to avoid dizziness or falls.**

Dizziness can result from fatigue. When the person you are caring for is rising from bed, remind him or her to sit on the bedside and dangle the feet and legs for a few minutes before standing up.

➤ **Plan regular activities.**

Plan an activity every day, even if it is as minor as getting dressed, walking out to sit on the porch, or taking a short stroll. Sometimes just seeing the sunlight or being in fresh air can help.

➤ **Serve regular meals as well as snacks.**

Serve a well-balanced diet with foods from the four basic food groups: grains (bread, cereal, rice, and pasta); fruits and vegetables; dairy products (milk, ice cream, cheese, and yogurt); and proteins (meat, poultry, fish, dry beans, eggs, and nuts). Call a community meals program, if necessary, to deliver balanced meals. Nutritious snacks add much-needed calories to the diet, and smaller portions of food served every few hours also help decrease fatigue.

Promote rest and sleep

➤ **Encourage as much activity as possible during the day so that normal fatigue sets in at night.**

➤ **Encourage a regular schedule of rest and sleep.**

Even a healthy person functions best when following a regular schedule of sleep. A regular schedule of naps and bedtimes is a great help in reducing fatigue in persons with HIV/AIDS.

➤ **Help reduce anxiety.**

Anxiety can interrupt rest and sleep. Talking, touching, and listening often help the person to manage this problem. For more suggestions on how to reduce anxiety, read the home care plan "Coping with Anxiety" (Chapter 18).

➤ **Encourage earlier bedtimes, sleeping later, and naps, as needed.**

If the person you are caring for is already taking naps regularly, then encourage longer naps to allow more rest and to reduce fatigue.

➤ **Play relaxing music or a relaxation tape before sleep.**

Music or the sound of the ocean or the television (on low volume) can be very soothing just before bedtime. Reading aloud to the person you are caring for may also be relaxing. Try whatever methods helped to promote sleep before.

➤ **Run a fan at bedtime.**

The constant, gentle whirring sound of a fan is relaxing and helps block out other noise.

➤ **Offer warm milk at bedtime.**

Warm milk can be soothing, and it contains nutrients that relax tired muscles.

➤ **Discourage spending too much time in the bedroom.**

Discourage eating, reading, watching TV, and visiting with friends while in bed. Try to keep the bedroom a place associated only with *sleeping*.

➤ **Give a warm bath or back rub at bedtime.**

Warm baths and back rubs relax aching, tense muscles and will help the person you are caring for to fall asleep.

➤ **Discuss sleep medicines with the physician.**

If you have tried all of the suggestions listed above and sleep remains a problem, ask the doctor if sleep medicine should be tried. *Do not give sleep medicine without checking with the doctor.* Some of these medicines should not be used in combination with other drugs. Be sure that the physician is aware of all other medicines that the person you are caring for is taking when you discuss whether sleep medicine should be prescribed.

4. POSSIBLE OBSTACLES TO CAREGIVING

Here are some common attitudes and misconceptions that may prevent you from carrying out your plan:

"Fatigue comes with the treatments. There's nothing I can do about it."

Response: Although some treatments of HIV/AIDS do result in fatigue, you *can* take steps to reduce fatigue and to control how it affects each day.

"There are so many things to worry about, it's no wonder I can't sleep."

Response: Help reduce anxiety in the person you are caring for. The home care plan "Coping with Anxiety" (Chapter 18) provides several suggestions on how to reduce worrying and make sleep easier.

Think of other obstacles

Identify additional roadblocks that could keep you from following the recommendations in this home care plan:

• Will the person I am caring for cooperate?

• Will other people help?

• How can I explain my needs to others?

• Do I have the time and energy to carry out this plan?

You need to develop plans for getting around these roadblocks. Use the four COPE ideas (Creativity, Optimism, Planning, and Expert information) in developing your plans. See pp 4–8 for a discussion on how to use the four COPE ideas in overcoming your obstacles.

CARRYING OUT AND ADJUSTING YOUR PLAN

Checking on results

Keep track of how much time the person you are caring for spends in bed. Pay attention to which recommendations for reducing fatigue are working and keep a list of what helps. Make certain that the most important or most enjoyable activities are done.

What to do if your plan does not work

1. Review this chapter.

2. If you find that you've skipped something, try it now.

3. If you find that you've done all that you can, call the doctor for further guidance.

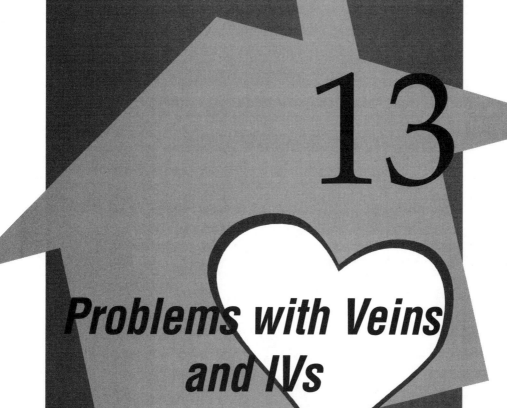

13

Problems with Veins and IVs

Overview of the Home Care Plan for *Problems with Veins and IVs*

1. *UNDERSTANDING THE PROBLEM*

> Types of intravenous (IV) devices
>
> Your goals

2. *WHEN TO GET PROFESSIONAL HELP*

> Symptoms that indicate the need for professional help
>
> Information to have ready when you call
>
> What to say when you call

3. *WHAT YOU CAN DO TO HELP*

> Prepare the skin and veins for needle sticks
>
> Limit discomfort and anxiety during needle sticks
>
> Learn about alternatives to needle sticks

4. *POSSIBLE OBSTACLES TO CAREGIVING*

5. *CARRYING OUT AND ADJUSTING YOUR PLAN*

> Checking on results
>
> What to do if your plan does not work

Topics that have an arrow (➤) in front of them are actions you can take or symptoms you can look for.

Problems with Veins and IVs

1. UNDERSTANDING THE PROBLEM

Many patients with HIV/AIDS need to receive intravenous (IV) medicines—that is, medicines administered directly into a vein. If a medication does not need to be given very often—for example, once per week—a single injection can be administered each time. If, however, the medicine needs to be given a few times each day over a period of a few days, a small plastic tube can be inserted in a vein and kept in place for 3 or 4 days at a time. Usually this IV tube is inserted in a vein in the hand. For people who need IV medications for longer periods, other intravenous devices are used. Blood tests are also often done to check the condition of the person with HIV/AIDS and to check the effects of medicines.

This home care plan will help you to understand the various IV devices and to know the symptoms to watch for that indicate the need for professional help, and will teach you how to help the person with HIV/AIDS care for arm veins and limit the anxiety and discomfort caused by blood testing.

> ➤ The information in this home care plan fits most situations, but yours may be different.
>
> ➤ If the doctor or nurse tells you to do something else, follow what he or she says.
>
> ➤ If you think there may be a medical emergency, see the section "When To Get Professional Help" on pp 144–145.

YOUR GOALS
Know when to call for professional help
Prepare skin and veins for needle sticks
Limit discomfort and anxiety during needle sticks
Learn about alternatives to needle sticks

2. WHEN TO GET PROFESSIONAL HELP

Symptoms that indicate an emergency

Call the doctor, nurse, or "after hours" phone number *immediately* if any of the following occurs:

➤ **Aching, tenderness, swelling, or redness (particularly a red streak) at the site of a needle stick (venipuncture) or an IV.**

These signs may mean that the skin or vein is reacting adversely to the drug or is infected. The arm or vein may need to be inspected by a health care professional. A health care professional can also tell you how to treat the problem (for example, using warm compresses).

➤ **Any drainage, pus, or blisters at the site of a needle stick or an IV.**

Clear or yellow-colored liquid that oozes from the needle stick site may be an indication of infection. Blisters also should be reported. If blisters contain any fluid, they should not be broken open.

➤ **The person you are caring for is so upset or nervous about needle sticks that he or she is considering skipping treatments or blood tests.**

Some people become so anxious about having blood drawn that they refuse to undergo treatments or blood tests. Heath care professionals know how to decrease anxiety about venipuncture. *Address this problem early so that important treatments are not missed.*

When you call, have the answers ready to the following questions:

1. When did the problem start?
2. Where are the veins that are sore?

3. When was the needle stick done or the IV inserted at the sites that are sore?

4. Is there a dark (black or blue) bruise?

Here is an example of what you might say when calling for professional help:

"I am Joan Smith, Harry Smith's caregiver. Harry is Dr. Brown's patient. Harry's skin is puffy at the injection site. An IV treatment was given yesterday at 2:00 P.M., and he noticed these problems when we got home at 5:00 P.M. What should I do?"

WHAT YOU CAN DO TO HELP

HERE ARE THREE STEPS YOU CAN TAKE:

Prepare the skin and veins for needle sticks

Limit discomfort and anxiety during needle sticks

Learn about alternatives to needle sticks

Prepare the skin and veins for needle sticks

It is often helpful to enlarge the veins so that they can be seen easily by whomever is going to perform the needle stick. The skin, too, can be prepared in such a way that the needle stick goes as smoothly as possible. Here are some ways of preparing the skin and veins for needle sticks:

➤ **Stay warm.**

Warmth makes the veins relax and fill up with blood. Sometimes a nurse will wrap the arm in a warm, wet cloth a few minutes before an injection. This helps the veins to dilate.

➤ **Eat and drink well the day before the treatment.**

Food and fluids help to maintain good blood flow through the veins. On the day of treatment, the person you are caring for should eat and drink normally, unless fasting (not eating anything) is required.

> **Drink 2 to 3 quarts of liquid every day, if possible.**

Fluids dilate or inflate the veins. Blood flows better, and the veins are more likely to stick up and be found easily. The person you are caring for should drink as much as possible, unless fluids are restricted for other reasons (for example, heart disease).

> **Take a walk immediately before chemotherapy or a blood test.**

Walking to the clinic or strolling around the clinic area just before the test or treatment helps to increase good blood flow and keeps the veins enlarged.

> **Exercise the hands and arms at home.**

Exercising at home can help makes veins bigger. Encourage the person with HIV/AIDS to squeeze a rubber ball or lift small weights (for example, cans of soup). He or she can do this while talking with family or friends or while watching television.

> **Use moisturizing lotions.**

The person you are caring for should apply a favorite lotion, cream, or ointment to the skin from fingertips to elbows. Lotion keeps the skin moisturized, which prevents dryness, cracking, and thickening of the skin. When the skin is dry, it is harder and more painful to puncture with a needle. The best time to apply moisturizers is after the skin has been wettened—after bathing, showering, swimming, or washing dishes. The skin should be patted *almost* dry before lotion is applied. Encourage the person you are caring for to do this as often as possible, at least four times each day.

Limit discomfort and anxiety during needle sticks

Venipunctures, or needle sticks, make many people anxious. Here are several ways of reducing or minimizing anxiety:

> **Remember or talk about pleasant experiences while waiting.**

Encourage the person you are caring for to talk and think about pleasant experiences just before a treatment or a blood test. Reading an interesting magazine or talking with another patient about something pleasant can also take his or her mind off the treatment. When the nurse is ready to perform the needle stick, the person you are caring for should try talking to the nurse (about something other than the needle stick) for distraction.

> **Remind the person you are caring for to "look away from the arm" during the test or treatment.**

Looking somewhere else in the room helps distract attention from the needle stick.

➤ **Talk to the doctor or nurse about the anxiety.**

The doctor may prescribe a medicine to make the person more relaxed or may recommend a mental health professional to help with these feelings. (See the home care plan "Coping with Anxiety" [Chapter 18] for more suggestions.)

➤ **Encourage deep breathing and other relaxation techniques during IV treatments or needle sticks.**

Relaxation is a skill that improves with practice. Encourage practicing relaxation techniques at home and using them before needle sticks. Ask the nurse to recommend books and tapes that teach deep muscle relaxation. (See the home care plans "Pain" [Chapter 14] and "Coping with Anxiety" [Chapter 18] for more suggestions on relaxation techniques.)

Learn about alternatives to needle sticks

If needle sticks are a continuing problem or if the person you are caring for needs to receive many of them over a long period, *try other ways of drawing blood for routine tests and other ways of administering drugs.* If you are interested in finding out more about these options, ask your nurse or doctor about them.

➤ **Regular IV: "Heparin Lock."**

These are very thin plastic tubes that are easily placed if the patient's veins are large enough. They can be used for approximately 3 to 4 days. Every time a medication is given through them, they must be "flushed" to keep them open for the next dose of medicine. Blood for tests cannot usually be drawn through this type of IV.

➤ **PICC (peripherally inserted central catheter) line.**

These are long, very thin tubes placed in a vein, usually in the arm, which then pass into a large vein. These tubes can sometimes be used to draw blood for tests. A PICC is usually put in place by a trained professional while the patient is lying down. Sometimes two tiny tubes are stuck together so that two different medicines can be given at the same time. It is important that the site where the IV enters the skin is kept clean and covered, and is watched closely for any redness or soreness.

➤ **IV catheters that connect to large veins.**

These catheters are special small, flexible, and sterile tubes that can be threaded under the skin into a large vein in the chest. These can be kept in place for months, with the ends taped to the chest or arm. These catheters, sometimes called Broviac or Hickman catheters, are used to draw blood for lab tests and to inject medicine or drugs used in chemotherapy into a large vein. The skin around the catheter is easily cleansed, and the site is not noticeable through clothing.

➤ Permanent ports or blood access devices.

Permanent ports are small (about 1 inch), round metal discs that are placed under the skin, usually on the chest. A small IV line extends from the permanent port into a large vein. It can be felt if you press lightly on the skin, but it is barely visible from the outside. A needle is pushed into the port site, and the drug is injected directly into the port.

➤ Finger sticks for some blood draws.

Sometimes a finger stick—a "pin prick" on the finger that gives only a drop or two of blood—is all that is needed for certain tests, such as a complete blood count (CBC) or platelet count.

➤ Ask about differences between IV catheters and permanent ports. Get answers to four important questions before choosing an IV option.

1. How often does the IV device, catheter, or port need to be flushed to stay open, and who will do this?

   Ports need to be flushed only once every 4 weeks if no drugs are given and no blood is taken. This usually takes about 5 minutes and can be done at a doctor's office or clinic. Visiting nurses can also do this at home if the person you are caring for is unable to travel. You, the person you are caring for, or family members may also learn to do this, but good control of the fingers and good vision is needed. A needle is pushed through the skin to get to the port underneath and is not usually painful.

   Intravenous catheters, such as a Hickman catheter, must be flushed every day to keep them open and available for future use. The dressing around them needs to be changed only three times per week. You or the person you are caring for may learn to do this, but good finger control and good vision are required. It is important to plan, in advance, *who should change these dressings, clean the skin around it, and flush the catheter every day.*

2. How much can a person move and exercise with an IV device, catheter, or port in place?

   Ports do not prevent athletic exercise because the port is under the skin. However, because catheters extend outside the body, swimming and some athletic sports are not advised, to prevent the catheter from being pulled out.

3. What does the treatment center recommend?

Some medical centers require that a certain catheter be used with certain drugs. If you know that the person you are caring for might be sent to a different medical center for treatment, ask which type that center prefers, and use the one they recommend.

4. Will the IV device, catheter, or port need more than one opening?

A "double"-opening port or catheter allows two different drugs to run into a large vein at the same time and allows for more treatment options.

POSSIBLE OBSTACLES TO CAREGIVING

Here are some common attitudes and misconceptions that may prevent you from carrying out your plan:

"The staff didn't say anything about ports or catheters, so I assumed they shouldn't be used."

Response: The health care staff may not know how upsetting needle sticks are to the person you are caring for. It is up to you to let them know. If it takes three or more attempts to perform needle sticks, you should ask about the availability and advisability of using ports or catheters.

"I've had trouble with needle sticks all my life, so nothing can be done."

Response: Health care staff members who give HIV/AIDS treatments are usually very experienced in performing needle sticks. They have had special training and understand how difficult this can be for some people. Therefore, you may find that needle sticks in an HIV/AIDS clinic are much less of a problem than you thought they might be. *Health care staff members are sensitive to this concern and will suggest ways to make the procedure as easy as possible.*

Think of other obstacles

Identify additional roadblocks that could keep you from following the recommendations in this home care plan:

• Will the person I am caring for cooperate?

• Will other people help?

• How can I explain my needs to others?

• Do I have the time and energy to carry out this plan?

You need to develop plans for getting around these roadblocks. Use the four COPE ideas (Creativity, Optimism, Planning, and Expert information) in developing your plans. See pp 4–8 for a discussion of how to use the four COPE ideas in overcoming your obstacles.

CARRYING OUT AND ADJUSTING YOUR PLAN

Checking on results

Watch for problems nurses or technicians have finding veins and whether the person with HIV/AIDS continues to be anxious about needle sticks. Pay attention to which recommendations are working, and keep a "diary" of your progress.

What to do if your plan does not work

1. Review this chapter.

2. If you find that you've skipped something, try it now.

3. If you find that you've done all that you can, call the doctor for further guidance.

14

Pain

Pain

14

Overview of the Home Care Plan for *Pain*

 1. *UNDERSTANDING THE PROBLEM*

Controlling pain

Types of pain

Your goals

 2. *WHEN TO GET PROFESSIONAL HELP*

Symptoms that indicate an emergency

Symptoms that may indicate an overdose or an allergic reaction to pain medication

Information to have ready when you call

Symptoms that do not indicate an emergency but should be reported

Symptoms that indicate severe pain

Information to have ready when you call

What to say when you call

 3. *WHAT YOU CAN DO TO HELP*

Make the best use of pain medicines

Understand the medication plan

Ask the doctor about changing prescriptions

Manage common side effects of pain medicines

Supervise pain management

 4. *POSSIBLE OBSTACLES TO CAREGIVING*

 5. *CARRYING OUT AND ADJUSTING YOUR PLAN*

Checking on results

What to do if your plan does not work

> **Topics that have an arrow (➤) in front of them are actions you can take or symptoms you can look for.**

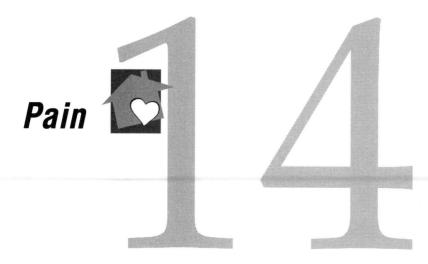

Pain

1. UNDERSTANDING THE PROBLEM

Pain is a common problem for persons with HIV/AIDS. Poorly managed pain limits a person's ability to engage in activities and affects quality of life. The good news is that pain can be controlled. Pain control can be accomplished through any of several measures, one of which is the use of effective pain medication. It often takes time to achieve satisfactory control of pain. It takes time for pain medication to build up in the body. The doctor may need to try different medicines or amounts to see what works best. Also, the pain control methods you and the person with HIV/AIDS can try take time to learn. Do not give up hope if pain control does not happen immediately. Eventually, almost all pain can be controlled.

There are two kinds of pain: acute and chronic. **Acute pain** is severe, is usually located in one area of the body, and may occur only occasionally. Acute pain may be a sign of a serious problem that should be reported. **Any new severe pain should be reported** *immediately*. **Chronic pain** is usually less intense, is always present, and often grows worse at night, when daily activities are no longer distracting

> ➤ The information in this home care plan fits most situations, but yours may be different.
>
> ➤ If the doctor or nurse tells you to do something else, follow what he or she says.
>
> ➤ If you think there may be a medical emergency, see the section "When To Get Professional Help" on pp 154–157.

the person from the pain. Although many persons with HIV/AIDS have both acute and chronic pain, this home care plan focuses on how to deal with chronic pain.

Pain medicines for chronic pain should be given regularly to prevent pain from building up. **It is much easier to prevent pain by using medicines regularly than it is to treat or reduce pain** *after* **it occurs.**

It is important that everyone be open and supportive to the person who is experiencing pain. Only the person who is in pain knows how much pain he or she is feeling. If the person who is in pain believes that others do not believe him, controlling the pain will be even more difficult.

YOUR GOALS

Know when to call for professional help

Make the best use of pain medicines

Understand the medication plan

Ask the doctor about changing prescriptions

Manage common side effects of pain medications

Supervise pain management

---

2. WHEN TO GET PROFESSIONAL HELP

Symptoms that indicate an emergency

These symptoms may indicate an overdose or an allergic reaction to pain medications.

If any of the following symptoms occurs while the person you are caring for is taking pain medications, call the doctor, nurse, or "after hours" phone number *immediately.*

➤ **Hallucinations (hearing or seeing things that are not present)**

➤ **Confusion or a feeling of being unaware of what is happening**

➤ **A drastic change in behavior**

➤ **Extreme dizziness, lack of balance, or inability to get up**

➤ **Inability to urinate despite feeling the need to do so**

➤ **Very slow, irregular breathing with periods of no breathing during sleep**

➤ **Hives, itching, skin rash, or swelling of the face**

➤ **Chest pain**

➤ **Shortness of breath**

➤ **Great trouble waking up or inability to wake up**

Call 911 immediately if you cannot awaken the person you are caring for. (Usually before such an incident occurs, you will have noticed a change in the person's level of alertness.)

When you call, have the answers ready to the following questions:

1. What pain medications were taken over the last few days?

2. How much medicine was taken?

3. How often has it been taken?

4. What *other* medications (prescribed or over-the-counter), if any, were taken? (For example, anti-anxiety medications, anti-depressants, anti-seizure medications, anti-nausea medications, cough medicines, anti-histamines, or cold and flu medicines.)

5. Were any "alternative treatments," herbs, or "special" remedies used?

6. Has he or she used alcohol or any recreational drugs recently or in the past?

Symptoms that do not indicate an emergency but should be reported during regular office or clinic hours

Some symptoms are not an emergency but should be reported during regular office or clinic hours. Call the doctor or nurse if any of the following symptoms occurs:

➤ **No relief 24 hours after taking pain medicine as prescribed.**

Ask if the dosage needs to be increased or if the person you are caring for should try a different medication. Also, a person with a history of heavy alcohol or recreational drug use may need a higher-than-usual dose of pain medicine to obtain good pain control if there is no relief after 24 hours.

➤ **"New" pain, pain in new locations, or pain when moving.**

New pains may need to be evaluated before the next regularly scheduled visit to the doctor because they usually indicate new problems which may need special treatment.

➤ **Numbness, tingling, or burning sensations.**

Numbness, tingling, or burning can signal a problem with the nervous system or with the types of medicine being taken. Report these symptoms early so that the doctor or nurse can determine what is causing them and make the necessary changes in the treatment plan.

➤ **Nausea with or without vomiting (which could be caused by pain medication).**

➤ **Constipation (which is often caused by pain medication).**

➤ **Inability to sleep because of pain.**

If the person you are caring for is unable to sleep because of pain, the pain is severe and needs to be treated.

➤ **The person you are caring for is crying and upset because of the pain.**

Look for physical responses to pain: tears, closed eyes, crossed eyebrows, wrinkled forehead, grimaced face, clenched fists, a stiffened trunk (chest and back) that is held rigidly, and slow movement (for example, while walking).

➤ **Unwillingness to move, tension in the muscles when moving, limping, or difficulty moving arms and legs.**

Even if the person you are caring for does not complain and tries to act as if nothing is wrong, watch how easily he or she moves. People in pain often try to avoid moving or doing everyday things (such as getting dressed and getting out of bed), or they move with great difficulty.

➤ **Decreased appetite.**

Watch for a sudden decrease in appetite. Although a diminished appetite can be caused by many other factors, do not rule out pain as the cause.

➤ **Withdrawal from family and friends.**

Pain can reduce the desire to visit with family and friends. Withdrawal from normal activities may also be a sign of depression, which may be caused by pain.

When you call, have the answers ready to the following questions:

1. How long has the person you are caring for been experiencing pain?

2. Where is the pain located? Is it located in more than one area?

3. How severe is the pain? Ask the person you are caring for to rate the pain on a scale of 1 to 10, where 0 = no pain, 5 = moderate pain, 10 = worst pain ever.

4. Is the pain sharp and stabbing or dull and aching?

5. Does the pain burn or feel like an electric shock?

6. Does he or she experience numbness or tingling?

7. How much has the pain interfered with normal activities?

8. What makes the pain worse?

9. Is he or she experiencing more than one type of pain at a time?

10. Describe any medication being taken for pain:

   How often should the medication(s) be taken (for example, every 4 hours)?

   How much medication should be taken at one time?

   How much medication has been taken during the last 2 days?

   How long does the medication take to work?

   How much relief does the medication give?

   How long does this relief last?

11. Have any methods other than medicine been tried to relieve the pain? What were the results?

Here is an example of what you might say when calling for professional help:

"I am Inez Vasquez, Isabelle Rosario's caregiver. Isabelle is a patient of Dr. Sanchez. I believe Isabelle is in severe pain. She avoids getting out of bed and walking around, and avoids even moving much at all. I see in Isabelle's face that she really hurts when she tries to get up from the bed or a chair."

3. WHAT YOU CAN DO TO HELP

HERE ARE FIVE STEPS YOU CAN TAKE:

Make the best use of pain medicines

Understand the medication plan

Ask the doctor about changing pain
 prescriptions, doses, and dosing intervals

Manage common side effects of pain medicine

Prevent and control pain on your own

If the pain is not an emergency, you can take some steps on your own to help relieve the pain.

Make the best use of pain medicines

If the person you are caring for needs medicine on a regular basis, *be sure that you are using the pain medicine correctly and preventing pain before it becomes severe.* The following suggestions will also help to relieve other problems that can increase pain, such as muscle tension, lack of sleep, and emotional distress.

➤ **Give the pain medicine at regular times, as prescribed by the doctor.**

When pain occurs regularly and not just once or twice a day, *give the pain medicine on a consistent schedule to keep enough medicine in the bloodstream to keep the pain away. Taking the medicine at regular intervals prevents "peaks and valleys" of pain by keeping a steady supply of the medicine in the body.* You may even find that you can decrease the *amount* of medicine given, because the person with pain is more confident that pain can be controlled.

Encourage the person you are caring for not to wait too long to take the medication. For example, if the doctor has instructed the person you are caring for to take the pain medicine "every 4 to 6 hours as needed," do not wait longer than 6 hours to give the medication. By that time, the pain may have become so severe that the prescribed amount will not give full relief—and it may also take longer for it to give *any* relief. A person who has pain needs to take pain medicine to avoid a pain crisis in the same way that a diabetic needs to take insulin to avoid a "sugar" crisis.

➤ **Continue to give pain medicine during the night.**

Try not to let more than 8 to 10 hours pass without giving medicine during the night, unless the person is taking a time-released

---

medicine such as MS Contin (a time-released capsule prescribed to be given every 12 hours). *As the time between doses becomes longer, the amount of medicine in the body decreases and the level of pain increases.* The person you are caring for will then need more of the medicine to return to a comfortable level because he or she will be below the "normal" medicine level at which good pain control is achieved. Giving pain medicine during the night helps to prevent what is called "breakthrough pain."

➤ **Do not discontinue pain medicine suddenly if it has been taken for several weeks.**

If pain medicine is discontinued suddenly, withdrawal symptoms may occur. The body has come to "expect" a steady flow of these medicines into the bloodstream. Withdrawal symptoms can occur in the same way that withdrawal occurs when a person suddenly stops smoking cigarettes or drinking coffee. The withdrawal symptoms may include shakiness or headaches.

If a pain medication needs to be discontinued, start by increasing the time between doses and by giving lower doses. This allows the body to be gently weaned from the medicines. Withdrawal symptoms are less likely if the pain medication is stopped slowly and *under the direction of a physician.*

Ask the doctor or nurse for answers to the following questions:

1. What should be done if the medicine wears off and the pain returns, but it is too early for the next dose?

2. If pain medicine is taken as prescribed but no relief from pain is achieved, can more medicine be taken without my needing to notify thedoctor?

3. What should I do if pain causes the person I am caring for to awaken during the night?

4. What should I do if a dose is accidentally skipped?

5. Can this medicine be crushed or can the pharmacist mix it in a liquid so that it is easier to swallow?

   (Some medicine, such as MS Contin, should not be crushed because this would prevent the medicine from being released at special times. This could be dangerous if the medicine is intended to be delivered in a time-released fashion.)

Understand the medication plan

Understanding how and when the doctor wants you to give pain medicines is the key to successful pain control and prevention. There are three possible plans. Ask the doctor which plan the person you are caring for needs to follow.

Plan 1: "Take medicine as needed" (or, "prn")

In this case, the patient must still take medicines *as prescribed* or as instructed on the label of the medicine bottle. For example, if the instructions read "take every 3 hours to 4 hours as needed," this means that the person you are caring for should *not* take the medicine *more often* than every 3 hours but is free to decide if he or she wants to take it less often (say, every 4 or 5 hours or more). He or she may wait until the first inkling of pain or until before beginning an activity that he or she knows will stimulate the pain problem. (Some people come to learn exactly what brings on pain, such as bending over the stove while cooking or bending to remove clothes from the dryer.) Taking pain medicine before these activities and then another dose 3 hours afterward may prevent the pain that sometimes follows. Again, encourage the person you are caring for not to let too much time pass between doses, because this will cause the level of medicine in the bloodstream to become too low and make the next dose less effective. If the person you are caring for finds that he or she needs the medicine more often than prescribed, this should be discussed with the doctor or nurse. Maybe the dose is not high enough, or maybe the medicine needs to be combined with another drug, such as Tylenol or aspirin, to prevent the pain. Keep track of how often (for example, recording the times in a notebook) the person you are caring for is taking the pain medicine and give this information to the doctor or nurse.

Plan 2: Take medicine at regular intervals

This means that the number of hours between doses should always be the same. If the doctor orders that the medicine be taken a certain number of times per day (such as two, four, or six times per day), start with the time that the person wakes up and divide the 24-hour day into equal parts. For example, if a medicine is prescribed to be taken "twice a day" and the person usually wakes up at 9:00 A.M., give one dose at 9:00 A.M. and the other at 9:00 P.M. Although the times do not have to be *exactly* right, you should try to divide the day into even sections as best you can. Other examples are as follows:

1. **The doctor orders that the medicine be taken "four times per day."** If the person you are caring for awakens at 9:00 A.M., give the first dose at 9:00 A.M., the second dose at 3:00 P.M., the third dose at 9:00 P.M., and the fourth dose at 3:00 A.M. (or some other time in the middle of the night).

2. **The doctor orders that the medicine be taken "six times per day."** If the person awakens at 9:00 A.M., give the first dose at 9:00 A.M., the second dose at 1:00 P.M., the third dose at 5:00 P.M., the fourth dose at 9:00 P.M., and the fifth and sixth doses at about 1:00 A.M. and 5:00 A.M., respectively.

Plan 3: Take medicine when pain "breaks through" before the next dose is due

"Breakthrough pain" is pain that returns before it is time for the next dose of pain medication. The doctor may prescribe something specifically for this breakthrough pain or may advise that an analgesic medicine be tried.

The first time that breakthrough pain occurs, make sure that the person you are caring for has been taking pain medicines consistently and as frequently as the prescription permits. Sometimes taking the pain medicine more consistently (that is, at regular intervals) and more frequently (for example, if the prescription reads "take every 4 to 6 hours," taking the medication every 4 hours around the clock) prevents breakthrough pain.

Ask the doctor about changing prescriptions, doses, and dosing intervals (the amount of time between doses)

➤ **Ask the doctor about switching to a different pain medication.**

This may be advisable if the person you are caring for is taking the medication as prescribed but is still experiencing significant pain or is bothered by side effects.

➤ **Ask about increasing the amount of medicine.**

Sometimes, there is just too little medicine in the body to prevent pain. If so, the doctor may increase the dose by small amounts until the right level of medicine in the body is achieved.

➤ **Ask about shortening the intervals between doses.**

Perhaps the right amount of pain medicine is not being maintained in the bloodstream because the medicine is not being taken often enough. If so, then the doctor may shorten the time between doses so that the level of medicine in the body is increased. Do not do this on your own without talking first with the doctor. Always report how much time passed before the pain returned.

➤ **Ask about adding other medicines.**

The doctor may combine several types of pain medicines that work in different ways to give relief. For example, an anti-anxiety medicine or anti-depressant can be added to decrease emotional tension, which, in turn, improves pain control.

➤ **Ask about giving the same medicine in a new form or in a new way to make it work more effectively.**

Pain medication can usually be given in more than one way:

Tablets and liquid pain medicine. If the person you are caring for cannot eat solid food, he or she may have trouble swallowing tablets. Some pain medicines are available in liquid form. The pharmacist may also be able to mix a liquid syrup with one or more pain medicines in it that can be given with a measuring spoon.

Skin patches. A recent invention is the transdermal patch; this patch is placed on the skin to deliver medicine through the skin for as long as 72 hours.

Rectal suppositories. Once placed in the body, the suppository melts and the pain medication is absorbed. Suppositories are very useful if the person you are caring for is nauseated or too weak to take pills.

Injections. Pain medicine can be received by injection into the muscle or just under the skin. If the idea of a long needle scares the person you are caring for, very short needles can be used. Many people who are not health care professionals can learn to give injections to family members or friends.

IV catheters. Some common IV catheters include Hickman, Broviac, and Groshong catheters, and catheters called PICC (peripherally inserted central catheter lines). These catheters are placed into large veins. The tubing runs to the outside of the skin for a few inches, with the medicine given in much the same way that it would be given through an IV line. These dressings are changed by nurses in the doctor's office or at home.

Epidural catheters. Catheters can also be placed around the spinal column to deliver pain medicine directly to the spinal fluid. Anesthesiologists can put epidural catheters in place near the spine to deliver medicines, and family members can then use these catheters to administer medicines.

Devices implanted under the skin. Implanted ports are another new way to deliver medicines through the larger veins of the body. Most ports are about 1 inch wide and 1 inch deep. The port is usually surgically placed under the skin in the upper chest. A catheter attached to it is placed in a large chest vein, allowing blood to be drawn and medicines to be given through the port.

IV infusion pumps. These are small, battery-operated pumps that can be carried in a pocket or on a belt. Infusion pumps deliver pain medicine around the clock in small, steady amounts through ports or IV catheters or both. If the patient is able to control the amount of pain medicine given through the IV infusion pump, it is called PCA—patient-controlled analgesia.

Sub-Q needles. A small needle can be placed just under the skin (called subcutaneous or Sub-Q) by a health care worker. This can be kept in place for about 3 days. Medicine is injected through this line every few hours (as directed) by a family member, or it can be hooked up to pumps that deliver the medicine at regular intervals. The needle must be changed and reinserted at a new site every few days by a nurse.

Manage common side effects of pain medicine

Although not all people react the same way to pain medicines, certain side effects are very common. Watch for these and deal with them early. The two most common side effects are drowsiness and constipation.

➤ **Prevent constipation.**

Because pain medicines decrease bowel activity and take water out of stools, constipation may occur. ***Constipation can be prevented by proper diet, stool softeners, and laxatives.***

Stool softeners are pills that put water back into stools, making them less hard and easier to pass. Taking one or two stool softeners in the morning and one or two at bedtime can also help *prevent* constipation.

In addition, mild laxatives, such as Metamucil and Citrucel, stimulate the bowels to move but should be used only after 2 days without a bowel movement. Another way to *prevent* constipation is to take Metamucil and Citrucel at night. These contain fiber, which is not digested in the stomach and small intestine. When fiber gets into the large (lower) intestine, it attracts water back into the intestine. This, in turn, softens the stool.

If stool softeners and laxatives do not help and the person you are caring for has not had a bowel movement in 2 to 3 days, talk with a health care professional. He or she may suggest a product that is a stronger laxative without a stool softener added, such as Milk of Magnesia, or that you increase the dosage of stool softeners or laxatives.

Other ways of preventing and alleviating constipation include the following:

1. Exercise, such as walking, prevents bowel activity.

2. Drinking several glasses of water each day (up to 2 to 3 quarts if the person with HIV/AIDS is not restricted to lower amounts because of previously diagnosed heart disease.) Water helps to soften the stool and make it easier to pass.

3. Eating foods high in fiber (for example, prunes, fresh fruits and vegetables, and foods containing bran).

Pain

14

> **Manage drowsiness.**

Sleepiness is likely to increase just after the person you are caring for starts or increases pain medicine, but later will decrease. *Sometimes sleepiness occurs because the person is finally getting pain relief and needs to catch up on missed rest. The body also needs time to adjust to new medicines or doses.* However, if sleepiness becomes a concern, offer beverages with caffeine in them, if allowed. Because pain medicines slow the responses somewhat, the way alcohol does, discourage the person you are caring for from driving a car, operating power tools, or any other activities that require fast reactions. If the drowsiness lasts longer than 3 days, contact the doctor so that the condition can be evaluated and corrected. *If drowsiness is extreme and you cannot awaken the person, call 911 immediately.*

Supervise pain management

> **Use a medicine box that helps "remind" the person about doses.**

"Medicine boxes" are plastic boxes with compartments for each day of the week. Larger-sized medicine boxes may have additional compartments to hold as many as four doses for each "day" compartment. Many people fill the box for an entire week ahead of time. If you can't find a plastic medicine box to suit your needs, an empty egg carton can work just as well; simply mark each slot with the name of the day of the week and the time that the pain medicine is to be given that day.

> **Set an alarm clock as a reminder to take pain medicines.**

> **Call the drug store before going to fill the pain prescription.**

Call before you try to fill the prescription. Some drug stores do not carry all pain medicines. They may have to special-order the medication you need or refer you to another store.

> **Use the same drug store regularly, if possible.**

Using the same drug store regularly will help the pharmacists understand what the medication plan is and how well it is working. This will also better enable them to answer your questions, to offer you suggestions on how to handle side effects, and to know what pain medication to keep in stock.

> **Keep at least a 3-day supply of pain medicines on hand.**

Call the doctor for a new prescription well in advance so that it can be called into a pharmacy or mailed to you in time. Be sure that you have at least a 3-day supply of pain medicine at all times—or, if it is the end of the week, a 5-day supply. If you are planning to be out of town, make sure you have a sufficient supply.

Practice other ways of controlling pain

In addition to giving pain medicines, you can help control pain several other ways:

➤ **Warm showers or baths, hot water bottles, heating pads, and warm washcloths.**

Heat relaxes the muscles and gives a sense of comfort. However, to avoid burning the skin, be careful not to set heating pads on "high" and make certain hot water bottles are wrapped in a cloth before they are applied to the skin.

➤ **Cool cloths.**

Cooling the skin and muscles can soothe pain, especially any pain that comes from inflammation or swelling. Applying a cool washcloth to the forehead is helpful in relieving a headache. However, do not use ice, because this can worsen the condition.

➤ **Position the person you are caring for carefully with pillows and seat cushions.**

Changing the person's position every 2 hours, when he or she is not able to do so himself or herself, will prevent muscle stiffness and painful pressure sores. Putting soft cushions on his or her chair will also prevent soreness.

➤ **Massage sore spots on the neck, shoulders, and tail bone.**

Massage and stretch the muscles in these areas to improve circulation and to prevent skin breakdown and soreness. Using some lotion for very short skin rubs (i.e., *less than 1 minute*) is advisable because it moistens dry skin. However, do not use lotion during the *longer* massage. It softens the skin too much and can make the skin break down.

➤ **Encourage deep breathing exercises.**

Deep breathing done slowly and quietly helps the mind and body to relax and thus helps decrease pain. Use relaxation tapes or learn simple methods from books on relaxation. Ask health care professionals about these techniques and read the home care plan "Coping with Anxiety" (Chapter 18) to learn more about relaxation.

➤ **Distract the person you are caring for with pleasant, involving activities.**

Pleasant activities can help distract the person you are caring for from the pain. Different activities work for different people. One person may be distracted by watching TV or looking through a catalog, while another may find listening to music or visiting with friends more effective. Plan activities for when the person you are caring for is most awake. This might be a few days after a new pain medicine is started or a few days after the dose has been increased. See the home care plan "Creating and Maintaining Positive Experiences" (Chapter 19) for additional ideas.

➤ **Keep a pain "diary" or calendar and rate the pain on a scale of 0 to 10, noting what makes it worse or better.**

Keep track of the times, amounts, and names of pain medicines given—and write down what makes the pain worse and what relieves it. This will help you judge what progress is being made. Bring this diary with you to doctor's appointments to keep the doctors and nurses informed about how the pain treatments are working.

➤ **Encourage the person you are caring for to avoid stressful events, when possible.**

Emotional stress and anxiety increase pain. If you can cancel or postpone events that you know will be very stressful, do so.

Be aware, however, that even pleasant activities can be stressful. Having fun requires energy. Resting before and after pleasant activities helps reduce the pain that flares up under stress.

 ## 4. POSSIBLE OBSTACLES TO CAREGIVING

Here are some common attitudes, fears, and misconceptions that may prevent you from carrying out your plan:

"I want to 'save' the pain medicine and take it when the pain is severe."

Response: Taking pain medicine "now" for mild discomfort does not affect how well it will work in the future, if or when the pain gets worse. There is no reason to "hold back" on pain medications in order to save them for a later time. The person you are caring for should be assured that he will not become "immune" to the pain medication and that the dose may need to be increased simply because the pain itself has changed or become more severe—not because he has become "immune" to the medicine.

If pain is controlled during the early stages of the disease, you and the person you are caring for will have more faith in your ability to control it later, as the disease progresses—which, in turn, will lessen anxiety. Taking enough medicine also keeps the person you are caring for from having to "fight" to get through each day. He or she will then be better able to conserve energy and stay encouraged.

"I don't want to become addicted."

Response: Sometimes people who are required to take morphine worry about becoming addicted. Taking morphine or other pain killers does not mean the person you are caring for will become an "addict." He or she is using pain medication to control pain, whereas an addict uses drugs to get high and abuses the amount that the doctor prescribes. People who take narcotics for pain rarely become addicted. He or she should not feel ashamed about using such drugs but should realize that they are a necessary part of the treatment plan.

"No one wants to hear about my pain."

Response: Family and friends may seem uninterested because they feel helpless, but they are actually very concerned. Be sympathetic when the person *does* talk about the pain. Doctors and nurses who specialize in pain, such as those who work in a pain clinic or hospice, do understand pain problems. Encourage the person you are caring for to talk to them if he or she is feeling alone with these problems.

"I don't want to take morphine, because only people who are close to death take that drug."

Response: Morphine is not reserved for the dying. It is a very effective medicine that is used for many types of pain, such as chronic pain during earlier stages of the disease. Some people go back to work and participate in their regular daily activities because the morphine is so effective. It allows them to resume pain-free lives.

Think of other obstacles

Identify additional roadblocks that could keep you from following the recommendations in this home care plan:

• Will the person I am caring for cooperate?

• Will other people help?

- How can I explain my needs to others?

- Do I have the time and energy to carry out this plan?

You need to develop plans for getting around these roadblocks. Use the four COPE ideas (Creativity, Optimism, Planning, and Expert information) in developing your plans. See pp 4–8 for a discussion of how to use the four COPE ideas in overcoming your obstacles.

CARRYING OUT AND ADJUSTING YOUR PLAN

Checking on results

Pay attention to which recommendations are working. Keep a "pain diary" (as discussed earlier in this chapter), by asking him or her to rate the pain regularly on a scale of 0 to 10 (where 0 = "no pain," 5 = "moderate pain," and 10 = "worst pain ever"). Report the pain levels to a doctor or nurse, especially if the levels are 5 or greater.

What to do if your plan does not work

1. Review this chapter.

2. If you find that you've skipped something, try it now.

3. If you find that you've done all that you can, call the doctor for further guidance.

Remember, pain can be well controlled. Do not accept anything less than the best pain control. If you feel that the medical staff are not listening to your concerns or are not able to give adequate pain control, you can ask to be referred to a pain specialist.

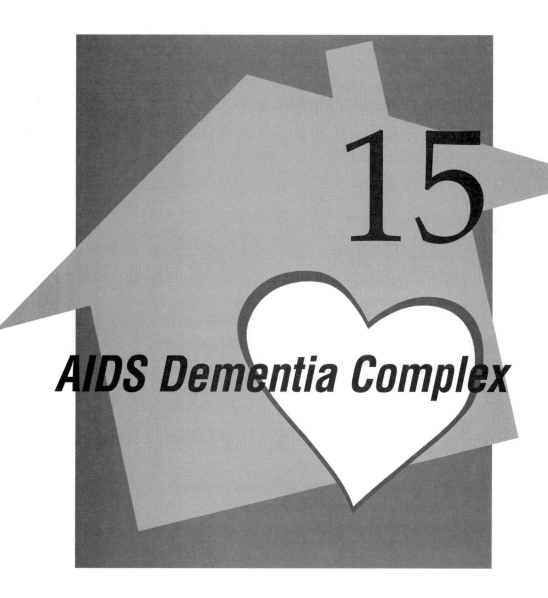

AIDS Dementia Complex

Overview of the Home Care Plan for
AIDS Dementia Complex

 1. *UNDERSTANDING THE PROBLEM*

What is AIDS dementia complex (ADC)?

Effects of ADC

Your goals

 2. *WHEN TO GET PROFESSIONAL HELP*

Symptoms that indicate the need for professional help

Information to have ready when you call

What to say when you call

 3. *WHAT YOU CAN DO TO HELP*

Provide a calm, stable home environment

Help the person you are caring for cope with a failing memory

Maintain a safe environment to prevent injuries

Set up an Advance Directive

 4. *POSSIBLE OBSTACLES TO CAREGIVING*

5. *CARRYING OUT AND ADJUSTING YOUR PLAN*

Checking on results

What to do if your plan does not work

Topics that have an arrow (➤) in front
of them are actions you can take or
symptoms you can look for.

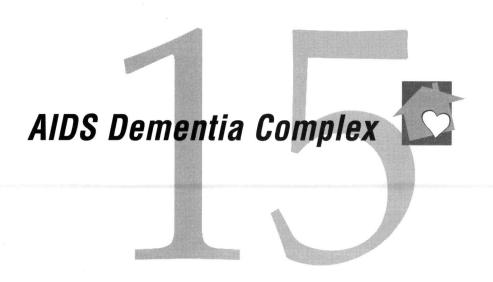

AIDS Dementia Complex

1. UNDERSTANDING THE PROBLEM

AIDS dementia complex—sometimes called ADC—is a common but difficult problem that may occur with HIV/AIDS. With ADC, the HIV virus damages the brain and nervous system, affecting thought processes, behavior, movement, and sensation. As the virus spreads within a person, ADC is more likely to develop. However, sometimes symptoms similar to ADC are *not* caused by HIV but by drug toxicities (too much of a medicine in the body).

Certain tests, such as computed axial tomography (CAT) or magnetic resonance imaging (MRI), can be used to diagnose ADC by showing changes in the brain. You, the caregiver, will see signs of ADC in the altered behavior of the person you are caring for.

As the thought processes are affected, the person with HIV/AIDS will have trouble with memory, concentrating, solving problems, and expressing thoughts completely, and may even be unaware of what is taking place around him. Personality changes can also occur. These differ from person to person but may include irritability, agitation, impulsiveness, and social withdrawal. The behavior of the person with ADC may resemble that of a depressed, mentally disturbed, or panic-stricken person. This is frightening both to the person with

> ➤ The information in this home care plan fits most situations, but yours may be different.
>
> ➤ If the doctor or nurse tells you to do something else, follow what he or she says.
>
> ➤ If you think there may be a medical emergency, see the section "When To Get Professional Help" on pp 172–174.

ADC and to those around him or her. Medications are available to help stabilize moods and behavior, which can help him or her to feel better and can make the home environment more peaceful.

Disturbances in movement may also appear. The person with ADC may become unsteady, uncoordinated, clumsy, and weak—especially in the legs. He or she may experience unpleasant sensations such as aching, burning, and numbness—again, primarily in the legs and feet—which affect walking. The person with ADC may have problems with movement and sensation in the hands, causing him or her to have difficulty writing, shaving, and handling utensils, and he or she may drop things frequently. All such changes should be reported to the doctor for evaluation.

This home care plan discusses ways of helping yourself and the person you caring for to cope with the changes that occur with ADC.

YOUR GOALS

Provide a calm, stable home environment

Help the person you are caring for cope with a failing memory

Maintain a safe environment to prevent injuries

Set up an Advance Directive

 ## 2. WHEN TO GET PROFESSIONAL HELP

Seeing the changes that occur with ADC can be very upsetting. As the disease progresses, symptoms that at first were barely noticeable will become very obvious. Reporting symptoms of ADC early is very important. Some medical conditions associated with the ADC are easily treated when diagnosed early. Also, health professionals can provide you with guidance about maintaining the safety and well-being of the person you are caring for.

Call the doctor or nurse if any of the following occurs:

> **Daily or new complaints of burning, tingling, and numbness in the hands and feet.**

These symptoms may be a sign that the AIDS virus has attacked the nerves in the body. However, certain medications may also cause burning, tingling, or numbness similar to that felt with ADC. If the condition continues without treatment, the person you are caring for may stop walking or using his or her hands. Report these problems before the condition becomes this severe.

➤ **Odd, abrupt changes in behavior or irrational behavior.**

The person you are caring for may begin to act or speak in a strange or nonsensical manner. He or she may even begin to have frightening and confusing hallucinations. The person may become irrational and cannot be reasoned with.

➤ **Depression, lack of motivation, or mood swings.**

The person you are caring for may seem depressed, lacking motivation and energy. You may also see the opposite form of behavior: irritability, excitability, anxiousness, and suddenly starting and stopping projects and tasks. He or she may also exhibit mood swings, in which a pleasant mood may quickly change to an irritable mood for no apparent reason.

➤ **Changes in vision, "staring into space," inability to communicate or talk with others, or loss of bowel and bladder control.**

These symptoms may be caused by ADC but could also be from other causes.

➤ **Slow and confused thinking.**

If the person you are caring for begins making obvious errors when performing simple tasks such as shopping and cooking, this is a sign that thinking has become slow and confused.

➤ **If you or the person you are caring for are in danger because of behavior changes.**

Professionals can help you to make the right decisions about how to get the best care for the person with dangerous behavior. Sometimes they might suggest medications that sedate behavior or improve depressed moods. In other cases, they may recommend day care or transfer to a nursing home or special AIDS facility.

When you call, have the answers ready to the following questions:

1. Has the behavior of the person you are caring for changed over a short period of time (for example, over a period of a few days)?

2. Has he or she suddenly become a danger to himself or herself or to others?

3. Has his or her personality changed to the opposite of what it used to be? For example, is a formerly calm and pleasant person now angry, anxious, and easily disturbed? Do there seem to be specific fears or reasons for his or her personality change?

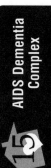

4. Are behavior changes accompanied by fever, headaches, changes in vision, or neck stiffness?

5. Does the person you are caring for require 24-hour supervision because it has become unsafe to leave him or her alone?

6. Has he or she recently started a new medicine or "alternative therapy"?

7. Has he or she begun falling or dropping things frequently?

8. Does he or she have great difficulty communicating or feel "lost" inside his or her own home?

9. Does he or she ever experience hallucinations?

10. Does he or she frequently wander out of the house?

11. Does he or she use recreational drugs?

12. Is he or she taking all medicines as prescribed?

13. What seems to help?

14. What seems to make things worse?

Here is an example of what you might say when calling for professional help:

"I am Betty Green, Jill Moran's caregiver. Jill is a patient of Dr. Becker. I have been noticing behavior changes in Jill. She is speaking and acting like a different person. Her thoughts are confused and her speech is sometimes scrambled. Often I can't even get her to understand what I'm saying. What should I do?"

3. WHAT YOU CAN DO TO HELP

HERE ARE FOUR STEPS YOU CAN TAKE:

Provide a calm, stable home environment

Help the person you are caring for cope with a failing memory

Maintain a safe environment to prevent injuries

Set up an Advance Directive

Provide a calm, stable home environment

➤ **Do not confront bizarre behavior in order to change it.**

Avoid arguments and confrontation. If the person you are caring for begins to show strange behavior or thought patterns, do not argue about them. Understand that those thoughts and behaviors are connected with the illness. *Stay calm, and gently help him or her to understand what is real and what is not. Do not feed into confused or irrational thinking by agreeing with it.* Instead, assure the person you are caring for that "everything is OK"and redirect his or her thinking to something that is soothing.

➤ **Keep the home as free of noise and agitation as possible.**

Noise, arguments, or any form of loud talking can cause a person who is feeling agitated or irritable to become even more so. Avoid inviting persons into the home who cause friction and arguments or who make the environment tense.

➤ **Establish set routines, and stick to them.**

The person who is experiencing confusion or agitation needs not only a calm environment but one that is free of changes. Set up a daily routine of activities and stick to it. He or she will come to know a fixed schedule of when to get up, when to eat, when to be involved in activities, and when to rest. The set schedule can keep the home setting stable at a time when the person is not feeling very emotionally stable.

➤ **Encourage the person you are caring for to make as many decisions on his own as he is capable of.**

A person with ADC is usually aware that changes in his or her behavior and feelings are occurring. The person may feel "out of control." Encouraging him or her to make decisions about his or her care will help the person regain some sense of control. Discuss decisions in the simplest manner possible, especially if you see that the person is confused. Discuss what the two of you will do step by step so that small goals can be met. This will boost morale and increase self-confidence.

Help the person you are caring for cope with a failing memory

If memory problems have occurred for the person with HIV/AIDS, you will probably see him or her making up stories or even telling lies to cover up the fact that he or she cannot remember. This problem is related to the AIDS dementia complex. Here are some steps that you can take:

➤ **Try to keep frequently used objects in the same place.**

We all know the frustration of misplacing or losing something that we need or use on a regular basis. Losing car keys, house keys, or eyeglasses can be exasperating, and much time can be wasted in repeatedly searching for them. Encourage the person with declining memory to put needed objects in the same place each time they are used. This will make them easier to find.

➤ **Use datebooks and calenders.**

Reviewing important dates, appointments, and holidays with a date book or calendar can help the person to remember scheduled events and appointments. A daily look at the calendar can also help the person to remember the day of the week, the month, and even the year.

➤ **Casually remind the person about the date, the time, and people's names.**

Such gentle reminders will help orient the person with a poor memory.

➤ **Keep the person you are caring for in touch with current events.**

Encourage the person you are caring for to watch the news on television or to listen to "news radio." You might also try reading newspapers or magazines aloud to the person if he or she finds it difficult to concentrate when reading. Sometimes just discussing current events will help him or her to stay "connected" with the world.

➤ **Encourage making lists of things to do or remember.**

Most people, including those without memory problems, find it helpful to make lists of things they want to remember—for example, shopping lists and lists of "things to do today." Encourage the person you are caring for to make such lists and place them in key places in the home, such as on the bathroom mirror, refrigerator door, or television set.

➤ **Gently remind the person you are caring for about how to perform everyday tasks.**

The person you are caring for may not remember how to do simple things like dress himself or herself or use the phone. If you see him or her faltering at such tasks, gently remind him or her what to do, step by step.

➤ **Help the person you are caring for to be honest about his or her memory loss.**

It is not unusual for a person with memory problems to lie or make up stories to cover up memory loss. (For example, he or she may claim to have fed the dog rather than admit to not remembering.) However, when such a pattern of lying is discovered it can cause arguments, frustration, and embarrassment. Help the person you are caring for to feel that it is acceptable to admit that his or her memory is poor at this time.

➤ **Encourage activities that stimulate the mind.**

Encourage the person you are caring for to read, to listen to the radio or watch television, or to talk with a friend. It is important that he or she avoid boredom and inactivity, because these cause the memory to decline even more.

Maintain a safe environment to prevent injuries

Safety should always be on your mind when the person you are caring for has ADC, because people with this condition are more likely to harm themselves because of poor judgment and loss of coordination.

➤ **Take measures to prevent falls.**

When the AIDS virus affects the nerves that control muscle movements, the person you are caring for will show signs of coordination problems. He or she may stagger, stumble, or fall frequently. You can create a safer home environment by removing obstacles and moveable objects that clutter or block the walking areas inside the home. Encourage him or her to use a walker or cane. Also, when going for a walk outside, make sure that the path that he or she will be taking is clear.

➤ **Monitor the safety of the person with ADC who smokes when alone.**

With ADC, movements can become jerky and uncoordinated. If the person you are caring for tries to smoke when no one else is present, self-harm and a fire within the home could easily occur. Therefore, set aside a special area for smoking where there are no materials that could catch on fire—for example, the front stoop of the house (provided that the stoop is concrete).

➤ **Assist the person you are caring for with his or her daily activities, as need dictates.**

Numbness, weakness, tingling, and tremors in the hands can interfere with the person's ability to prepare a meal, eat, shave, dress, and even bathe. Provide assistance, when needed, while still encouraging the person's independence and self-care as much

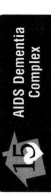

AIDS Dementia Complex

as possible. Consult the nurse, social worker, or occupational therapist about purchasing or borrowing devices that can help with cooking, eating, or bathing. Adjustments can be made on clothing, such as Velcro instead of buttons or zippers, to allow for self-care.

➤ **Encourage remaining as active as possible.**

The person with ADC who is experiencing uncoordinated muscle movements and unpleasant sensations in the hands and feet may tend to stay in bed more and to do less. This can cause additional problems, including boredom and depression, bedsores, increased weakness, and increased risk of respiratory infections. You should encourage the person you are caring for to remain as active as possible. If pain or tingling causes inactivity, look into obtaining pain medications for relief.

➤ **Supervise use of medicines.**

If the person with ADC has memory problems, you will need to help him or her to remember to take medications on schedule. Setting up the medications for him or her, posting reminders around the home, or using an alarm clock to signal medication times may help. You may also need to control the medication supply, dispensing small amounts of medicine for certain hours of the day. Throughout the day and night, you may have to check periodically to make sure that the person is not in pain. See the home care plan "Pain" (Chapter 14, pp 158–165) for more suggestions on supervising use of medications.

Set up an Advance Directive

If the person you are caring for has ADC, he or she may not be able to make decisions near the end of his or her life. Therefore, an Advance Directive should be set up before the ADC becomes severe. An Advance Directive is a *living will*, which clearly states the person's wishes about medical treatment at the end of life and about who should have the *health care power-of-attorney*. This "attorney" is an individual selected by the person with HIV/AIDS—usually a family member or close friend—who makes decisions about medical matters in the event that the person with HIV/AIDS cannot. *Ask a nurse, social worker, or doctor about getting the paperwork to complete an Advance Directive form.*

4. POSSIBLE OBSTACLES TO CAREGIVING

Here are some common attitudes and misconceptions that may prevent you from carrying out your plan:

"Everyone forgets things from time to time. My memory is no worse than yours or anyone else's."

Response: It is easy for the person with ADC to want to brush aside or cover up signs that his or her ability to think is impaired. Help him or her to understand that forgetfulness and confusion can cause other serious problems, such as falls, fires, or forgetting to take medicine, and should not be ignored. Perhaps mention consequences of these events and describe how they would make the situation harder for both of you.

"I don't need that cane (or walker). I think you're being overprotective. I just fell a few times. Those things are for old people. I wouldn't leave the house with one of them."

Response: Help the person you are caring for to accept that these devices will help keep him safe from falls and broken bones, and will actually help him remain more active and independent, rather than make him more like an "invalid" or an "old person." You might say something like, "It will help me to know you are as safe as possible. Could you do this for me?"

"You say that I'm acting differently lately. Maybe I do fly off the handle a bit, but most people do. Besides, don't you think I have reason to get upset or anxious?"

Response: You might respond by saying something like "Yes, I agree that you have reason to be upset, but I also want to be sure that nothing else is wrong." Instead of allowing the person you are caring for to see that you are frightened or disturbed by his or her behavior, report them to the physician and deal with the person gently, reasonably, and with understanding.

Remember, persons with ADC are not acting or thinking irrationally because they are lazy or want to irritate you. Try not to take their words or behavior personally as an attack against you.

Think of other obstacles

Identify additonal roadblocks that could keep you from following the recommendations in this home care plan:

- Will the person I am caring for cooperate?

- Will other people help?

- How can I explain my needs to others?

- Do I have the time and energy to carry out this plan?

You need to develop plans for getting around these roadblocks. Use the four COPE ideas (*C*reativity, *O*ptimism, *P*lanning, and *E*xpert

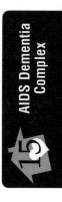

information) in developing your plans. See pp 4–8 for a discussion of how to use the four COPE ideas in overcoming your obstacles.

5. CARRYING OUT AND ADJUSTING YOUR PLAN

Checking on results

If the person with HIV/AIDS is less discouraged and frustrated, and is more calm and peaceful and able to look after himself or herself, you are on the right track. However, keep in mind that his or her condition may become worse through no fault of your own. Keep track of changes in symptoms and report them to the physician or nurse.

If your plan does not work

Watch for continued problems. Pay attention to which recommendations are working and keep a diary of your progress.

What to do if your plan does not work

1. Review this chapter.

2. If you find that you've skpped something, try it now.

3. If you find that you've done all you can, call the doctor for further guidance.

If the situation seems too hard to handle, do not hesitate to get professional help. There is no shame in admitting that you cannot continue to provide care without more assistance. Managing ADC is one of the most difficult parts of caring for someone with HIV/AIDS, and nearly everyone needs additional help.

16

Emotional and Social Stress Related to HIV/AIDS

Overview of the Home Care Plan for
Emotional and Social Stress Related to HIV/AIDS

 1. UNDERSTANDING THE PROBLEM

Emotional issues related to HIV/AIDS

Family reactions to the diagnosis of HIV/AIDS

Social stress and issues confronting persons with HIV/AIDS

Your goals

 2. WHEN TO GET PROFESSIONAL HELP

Symptoms that indicate the need for professional help

What to say when you call

 3. WHAT YOU CAN DO TO HELP

Deal with feelings of hopelessness

Confront anger

Cope with feelings of rejection and isolation

Help the person you are caring for to accept loss

 4. POSSIBLE OBSTACLES TO CAREGIVING

5. CARRYING OUT AND ADJUSTING YOUR PLAN

Checking on results

What to do if your plan does not work

> **Topics that have an arrow (➤) in front of them are actions you can take or symptoms you can look for.**

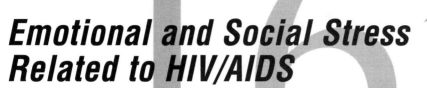

Emotional and Social Stress Related to HIV/AIDS

1. UNDERSTANDING THE PROBLEM

HIV/AIDS can cause some difficult emotional and social problems. Emotional problems may include fear; uncertainty about the future; anger at the disease, at self, and at health care staff; a sense of hopelessness and feelings of loss; and a struggle with guilt and shame.

Social problems include dealing with the responses or reactions of others to the diagnosis. For the family of the person diagnosed with HIV/AIDS, it may be the first time that they learn that a son or daughter is gay or an IV drug user. The family may feel shocked, angry, dismayed, or betrayed. Messages of disapproval can drive the person with HIV/AIDS into isolation and social withdrawal, and he or she may sever ties with important persons in his or her life.

The reactions of society to the diagnosis of HIV/AIDS may range from fear and rejection to moral self-righteousness. The person with HIV/AIDS, therefore, is dealing not only with his or her own emotional responses to the diagnosis but is confronted with society's often complex and sometimes differing opinions about the nature and cause of the disease.

> ➤ The information in this home care plan fits most situations, but yours may be different.
>
> ➤ If the doctor or nurse tells you to do something else, follow what he or she says.
>
> ➤ See the section "When To Get Professional Help" on pp 184–185.

> ## YOUR GOALS
>
> Know when to call for professional help
>
> Deal with feelings of hopelessness
>
> Confront anger
>
> Cope with feelings of rejection and isolation
>
> Face losses

2. WHEN TO GET PROFESSIONAL HELP

Dealing with social pressures as well as with the stress and emotional burden of having HIV/AIDS can be very difficult, sometimes leading the person who has the disease to adopt behaviors that are unhealthy and self-defeating.

Some people are hesitant to ask for help with emotional problems because they do not want to appear "crazy." They should understand that having emotional problems during a major illness is perfectly normal—and that getting help for these problems is normal, too. When seeking professional help, it is best to start with the doctor treating the disease, who is familiar with the person you are caring for and with the stage of his or her illness. Sometimes convincing the person with HIV/AIDS to get help is difficult, especially while he or she is upset. The best you can do is to use a loving, gentle approach and give a clear message that you care and that you think professional help is needed.

Mental health professionals (psychologists, psychiatrists, and social workers) are experienced in helping people with emotional problems. Many mental health professionals have experience treating people with HIV/AIDS and understand ways of treating emotional problems brought on by the stress of the illness. Signs that the person you are caring for requires professional help include the following:

➤ **The person you are caring for has broken ties with almost everyone he or she once knew and is rarely seen by others.**

Negative comments and reactions of family and friends can lead to feelings of guilt, worthlessness, and depression. Sometimes these feelings may arise even when family and friends are supportive. These feelings can be very crippling and may lead the person to quit fighting the disease. Also, withdrawing from others makes it impossible to for the person to receive the emotional support he or she needs. A health care professional or support group can often encourage the person you are caring for to look at and talk about his or her negative feelings, and ways of acquiring much needed acceptance and support can be discussed. The love and acceptance of others can be a powerful force in motivating the person to seek wellness.

➤ **The person you are caring for has become so angry and resentful that he or she refuses needed medical care or is violent or threatening.**

Anger toward self or toward the disease can easily be directed at those who are helping to treat it. For example, it is not unusual for a person with HIV/AIDS to complain about the doctor or the clinic where he or she goes for treatment. Because small health problems can easily turn into larger ones, anger and feelings of helplessness can cause the person with HIV/AIDS to stop treatment altogether. He or she may feel that medical care is not adequate or proper. This may or may not be true but should be discussed openly with health care professionals. Any threats to others or against himself or herself, such as angry threats to commit suicide, should also be reported to health care professionals. The safety of everyone involved is very important.

➤ **The person you are caring for is depressed or is contemplating suicide.**

The emotional strain of facing the reactions of others and of combating one's own fears about the disease can make persons with HIV/AIDS feel very hopeless. When this happens, depression or despair can easily set in, blocking the desire to fight the disease and live. The person you are caring for may lose a sense of purpose and meaning in life. This can occur as early as when the diagnosis is first made, or it may be later during the course of the illness. If you see signs of depression, contact a health care professional *before* the person you are caring for begins to contemplate or attempt suicide. (For more discussion of the symptoms of depression, see "When To Get Profession Help" on pp 196–198 of the home care plan "Coping with Depression," Chapter 17.)

➤ **The person with HIV/AIDS reacts to stress or expresses anger by physically abusing you, other caregivers, or health professionals.**

Your safety and the safety of others who are helping are extremely important. *Get professional help immediately if you or others are in danger!*

Here is an example of what you might say when calling for professional help:

"I am Maria Diaz, the caregiver of Rodrique Diaz. Rodrique is a patient of Dr. Blackwell. Rodrique has not been doing well since he had pneumonia 2 months ago. He keeps saying that his disease is getting out of control, and that he therefore should no longer bother seeing Dr. Blackwell for treatment. He keeps saying that nothing will help. I don't believe that, but I can't convince him that things can get better. What should I do?"

3. WHAT YOU CAN DO TO HELP

> ### HERE ARE FOUR STEPS YOU CAN TAKE:
>
> Deal with feelings of hopelessness
>
> Confront anger
>
> Cope with feelings of rejection and isolation
>
> Face losses

Deal with feelings of hopelessness

Hopelessness and depression are usually intermingled. For a more full discussion of depression, see the home care plan devoted to this topic, "Coping with Depression" (Chapter 17).

➤ **Encourage talking openly about the feelings that are causing the hopelessness.**

Poor self-esteem or even self-hate can get in the way of attempts to get well or attempts to remain optimistic about the future. Encourage the person to talk openly with a trusted friend or loved one about such feelings, if they exist. If self-hate is the problem, talking with a clergyman or professional counselor may be necessary.

Talking about such feelings with trusted friends, clergymen, or mental health professionals can help the person you are caring for to begin to forgive himself or herself as well as to forgive those who do not understand, who are not accepting, or who cannot be supportive.

➤ **Encourage the person you are caring for to take responsibility for his or her own life.**

Blaming oneself, others, circumstances, God, or fate for one's present situation is easy to do. Taking responsibility for one's own life and for how it will be lived from this moment forward is more difficult but more rewarding. Taking control means being in charge of what happens. It means fighting to get well and stay well. It also means remaining optimistic.

➤ **Encourage staying involved in meaningful activities.**

It is important that the person you are caring for continues working or staying involved in normal, daily activities for as long as possible. This will bolster self-esteem and feelings of worth. Being involved in some form of everyday routine, such as having meals with others, can bring meaning to each new day and make it less easy to step into the "sick role."

➤ **Set goals for each day.**

Setting goals for each new day and discussing how these goals can best be met will give the person you are caring for something to look forward to, provide a sense of accomplishment, and help him or her to live one day at a time.

Confront anger

Although anger is a natural response to unfair events or circumstances, it may lead a person to focus on negative and resentful feelings. Anger directed at oneself can lead to depression. Anger can also sometimes cover up other feelings that a person does not want to acknowledge. It is important to try to discover the reasons for anger and to learn which are the best ways of dealing with it.

➤ **Identify the sources of anger.**

The person you are caring for may be angry at himself or herself for contracting the disease or at the disease itself for changing his or her life so greatly. He or she may also be angry at family members or friends who may not be understanding, accepting, or available, or at health care professionals who seem to be unhelpful. Progression of the disease and the prejudice of others toward people with HIV/AIDS are other causes of anger. Feelings of panic, uncertainty, helplessness, denial, or hopelessness can also lead to anger.

When the person you are caring for can pinpoint why he or she is angry, the anger will be easier to deal with. Expressing these feelings by crying, sulking, raging (in a manner that does not hurt oneself or someone else), discussing them with a friend, or writing about them also makes it easier to deal with the anger.

➤ **Discover positive ways of releasing anger.**

Some people have found that anger can be released through physical activity, such as swimming, running, cleaning, or doing yard work. Other people are more comfortable with releasing anger through more gentle activities, such as writing about their feelings in a journal, talking about their feelings with a friend, or crying. One can "talk out" anger while looking into a mirror or can "scream it out" in an isolated place. Relaxation or meditation can also be helpful in dealing with anger. See the home care plan "Coping with Anxiety" (Chapter 18) for a discussion on relaxation techniques. The final goal of all of these activities, and perhaps the hardest, is to be able to forgive oneself as well as forgive others. Forgiveness helps one to let go of pain, resentment, and anger, and to feel free.

➤ **Help the person you are caring for accept what cannot be changed.**

Anger can be a good motivator for examining one's situation and making necessary changes. However, some circumstances, such as having HIV/AIDS, will not change. Acceptance of reality and working within it are necessary. *Acceptance does not mean giving up.* It means adapting and moving forward.

Cope with feelings of rejection and isolation

Having an illness such as HIV/AIDS may mean facing rejection by friends, family, and society. To avoid any possible rejection, the person you are caring for may try to isolate himself or herself.

The person with HIV/AIDS needs to deal with the pain of rejection by others. Here are some ways you can help:

➤ **Remind the person you are caring for that he or she needs support from others.**

Although isolating oneself may seem like the right thing to do when one is feeling rejected, this may only set off a process of self-pity. Staying connected with others and sharing thoughts and opinions can keep self-pity from occurring. It is far less frightening to face illness with others at one's side than it is to face it alone.

➤ **Encourage reaching out to those who care.**

It is very important that the person you are caring for have a group of persons on whom he or she can depend. The first step in reaching out for support is telling those people who can be trusted about having HIV/AIDS. This takes courage, as well as good judgment. *Not everyone needs to know.* Those who would be very upset or traumatized by having this information should not be told. After hearing about the diagnosis, some people will be taken by surprise, others will respect the honesty, and still others will be burdened and upset by the information. Such responses are to be expected. After the truth has been shared, those who recover more easily from the news will be the ones on whom the person can depend. Their assistance and support will be needed at each stage of the disease process. Initially, other people are needed primarily for encouragement and understanding, but as the disease progresses their *care* as well as their moral support will be needed.

➤ **Encourage getting support from those who have faced similar experiences.**

Support groups consist of persons with similar backgrounds, experiences, and problems. It is within such groups that persons with HIV/AIDS can feel truly accepted and understood. Group members share experiences that other group members can understand. Solutions to problems are discussed, and suggestions for coping are shared. All this takes place in an atmosphere of loving, caring, and support.

As a caregiver, you should encourage the person you are caring for to join such support groups. Support groups for the caregivers themselves have also been formed. You can ask a health care professional to refer you to any of the several support groups that now exist for persons with HIV/AIDS—or you can contact the AIDS National Interfaith Network for a referral (for more information, see Appendix A on p 307).

Help the person you are caring for to accept loss

Recognizing the many losses a person faces when coping with HIV/AIDS is important. The loss of health and well-being are two of those losses. Loss of self-esteem and respect can also be experienced. Loss of a sense of control over one's own life is strongly felt because of the uncertain nature and course of the disease. When illness places the person within the health care system, this "loss of control" is even more keenly felt. It may seem that decisions are being made about the person without his or her input. Because facing loss is painful, many people try to "block out" their feelings and thoughts—through denial and even drugs and alcohol. You can help the person you are caring for accept loss by trying the following suggestions:

➤ **Take steps similar to those used in dealing with anger.**

The first step is to identify what losses one has experienced. The second step is feeling and expressing the sadness connected with the losses. The third step is recognizing that what one has lost will not be regained.

The goal is for the person to let go of what he or she has lost and to hold on to what he or she still has. Bear in mind that this can be difficult, because many people feel that life will never be the same without what they have lost. They yearn for what was and can spend much energy on their regrets. They need to let go to move forward—to accept the losses and to go on with life, despite the losses. Help the person you are caring for to express grief over loss, by listening and by talking with him or her.

➤ **Help the person you are caring for accept the possibility of death.**

Every person who has a fatal illness such as severe heart disease, advanced cancer, and AIDS faces the possibility and fear of death. Some people become paralyzed by the fear of death early in their disease, allowing this fear to prevent them from enjoying the period of life that is theirs to have. Being able to live each new day to the fullest and to live "one day at a time" is a skill that people facing death need help in developing.

Not only the person with HIV/AIDS but also his or her caregivers, loved ones, family, and friends, need to face the reality of death. Talking openly and honestly about this reality and slowly preparing for it will allow death to be a more peaceful event. For more suggestions on how to face this hard reality and how to live life to its fullest, see the home care plans "Creating and Maintaining Positive Experiences" (Chapter 19) and "The Last Weeks of Life" (Chapter 24).

 ## 4. POSSIBLE OBSTACLES TO CAREGIVING

Here are some common attitudes and misconceptions that may prevent you from carrying out your plan:

"Talking about having HIV/AIDS just increases my stress and everyone else's. People are better off if they don't know."

Response: Initially, the news that a friend or loved one one has HIV/AIDS is shocking, saddening, and difficult to accept. At first, keeping this information from others may seem best. However, as the disease progresses, the person you are caring for will have to depend on the very people he or she does not want to tell. You can help the person you are caring for to carefully select who to tell about the diagnosis. More important, trusted people should be told before health problems become overwhelming.

"Of course I'm angry. Who wouldn't be? They make me take so many tests and treatments. The staff are always telling me what I should and shouldn't do."

Response: Anger at the disease of HIV/AIDS is easily directed at medical staff and caregivers. Remember that it is when people are feeling the most helpless that they seem to be the most resistant to help and become most angry. Helping the person with HIV/AIDS to talk about the fears, the uncertainties, and the help-lessness that he is expressing through angry words and mannerisms can help him to control his feelings. This is important for a good quality of life for him and for you.

Think of other obstacles

Identify additional roadblocks that could keep you from following the recommendations in this home care plan:

- Will the person I am caring for cooperate?

- Will other people help?

- How can I explain my needs to others?

- Do I have the time and energy to carry out this plan?

You need to develop plans for getting around these roadblocks. Use the four COPE ideas (Creativity, Optimism, Planning, and Expert information) in developing your plans. See pp 4–8 for a discusssion of how to use the four COPE ideas in overcoming obstacles.

5. CARRYING OUT AND ADJUSTING YOUR PLAN

Checking on results

Many strong feelings and reactions occur among family members, friends, and loved ones of a person with HIV/AIDS when they learn of the diagnosis. It is understandable that they feel shocked and sad. However, when honesty, love, and trust exist, loved ones will, in time, adjust and can be counted on to provide support and care. You will know that others have dealt with these issues when you see fam-ily and friends coming forward to help. You will know whether the person you are caring for is coping well when he or she expresses a sense of hopefulness and seems able to find meaning in life.

What to do if your plan does not work

Continue to give the clear message that you care, and follow these steps:

1. Review this chapter.

2. If you find that you've skipped something, try it now.

3. If you find that you've done all that you can, call the doctor for further guidance.

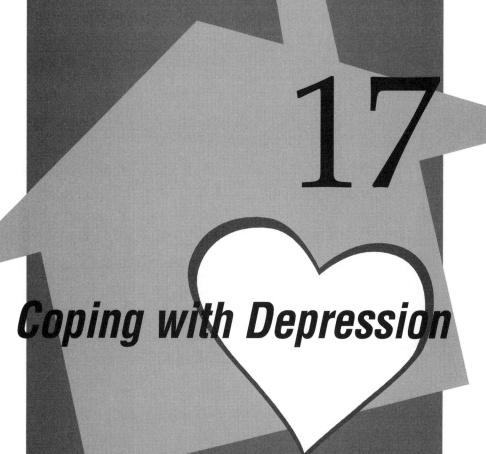

Coping with Depression

Overview of the Home Care Plan for
Coping with Depression

1. ***UNDERSTANDING THE PROBLEM***

> The cycle of depression
>
> The downward spiral of depression
>
> The effects of depression on both the person with HIV/AIDS and the caregiver
>
> The need for teamwork between the caregiver and the person with HIV/AIDS
>
> Your goals

2. ***WHEN TO GET PROFESSIONAL HELP***

> Symptoms that indicate the need for professional help
>
> What to say when you call

3. ***WHAT YOU CAN DO TO HELP***

> Take care of your own emotional needs
>
> Get professional help for yourself, if necessary
>
> Prevent or decrease depression

4. ***POSSIBLE OBSTACLES TO CAREGIVING***

5. ***CARRYING OUT AND ADJUSTING YOUR PLAN***

> Carrying out your plan
>
> Checking on results
>
> What to do if your plan does not work

6. ***TECHNIQUES FOR CONTROLLING NEGATIVE THOUGHTS***

> **Topics that have an arrow (➤) in front
> of them are actions you can take or
> symptoms you can look for.**

Coping with Depression

The person you are caring for is the one who will use the techniques outlined in this home care plan: Your job is to help him or her make the best use of these techniques. Have the person you are caring for read this chapter, and then the two of you should work together as a team. You, the caregiver, may also use the techniques discussed in this chapter if you find that you are depressed or discouraged.

1. UNDERSTANDING THE PROBLEM

Almost everyone has times of feeling discouraged or depressed. These feelings are normal and usually do not last too long, tending to "go away by themselves" or to diminish when the problem that causes them is resolved. The stress of dealing with a chronic illness

> ➤ The information in this home care plan fits most situations, but yours may be different.
>
> ➤ If the doctor or nurse tells you to do something else, follow what he or she says.
>
> ➤ See the section "When To Get Professional Help" on pp 196–198.

such as HIV/AIDS, however, can cause depression to persist for long periods. Sometimes lack of energy or simply not feeling well may bring on depression in the person with HIV/AIDS. The depression, in turn, may make it more difficult for the person to cope with his or her illness; he or she may become so trapped in negative feelings that it becomes too difficult to take actions toward getting well. The depression may become so severe that the person will contemplate or attempt suicide.

Depression works like a downward spiral. When a person is depressed, he or she may not put energy into solving problems. This causes the problems to become worse, which then causes the the person with HIV/AIDS to feel worse. And so on and so on. *This destructive pattern needs to be interrupted.* If the pattern is allowed to continue, it will become more and more difficult for the depression to simply "go away on its own."

This chapter discusses ways of helping the person who is depressed to cope. The caregiver's help and encouragement are important, but the person with HIV/AIDS must practice self-help strategies. You and the person with HIV/AIDS should work together as a team to deal with depression.

However, bear in mind that some depression is a normal response to the stresses and uncertainties of chronic illness. *Do not expect to get rid of all feelings of depression. Nevertheless, you can help to limit the duration and severity of depression.*

It is also important to remember that living with a person who is overwhelmed by illness, discouraged, or depressed can be stressful and discouraging to a caregiver. Pay attention to your own emotional health and well-being. The information in this home care plan can help you, too.

YOUR GOALS

Know when to get professional help

Take care of your own emotional needs

Get professional help for yourself, if necessary

Prevent or decrease depression

WHEN TO GET PROFESSIONAL HELP

Some people are hesitant to ask for help with emotional problems because they do not want to appear "crazy." They should understand that having emotional problems during a major illness is normal—

---

and that getting help for these problems is normal, too. When seeking professional help, it is best to start with the doctor treating the disease, who is familiar with the person you are caring for and with the stage of his or her illness.

You can also call mental health professionals, such as psychologists, psychiatrists, and social workers, all of whom are experienced in helping people with emotional problems. Many mental health professionals have experience treating people with HIV/AIDS and with depression that is brought on by the stress of the illness.

Signs that the person you are caring for requires professional help include the following:

➤ **The person you are caring for is contemplating suicide.**

Anyone who talks about committing suicide should be taken seriously. If the person you are caring for is not openly *talking* about suicide but you suspect that he or she is nevertheless *thinking* about suicide, ask him or her about it. Asking will not make it more likely.

If the person you are caring for is considering suicide, *you should get professional assistance as soon as possible.*

➤ **The person you are caring for has suffered from serious depression that required professional help before this illness and is now feeling depressed again.**

Anyone with a history of serious depression is vulnerable to depression after a major life stress. A serious illness such as HIV/AIDS often triggers depression in these people. Professional help is usually required.

➤ **The person you are caring for has had at least two of the following signs of depression consistently during the past 2 weeks:**

Feelings of sadness most of the time

Loss of concentration

Loss of interest or pleasure in things or activities that were once enjoyable

Increase or decrease in appetite

Change in sleep patterns

Feelings of self-blame and guilt

Low self-worth

Tearfulness

Irritability

➤ **The person you are caring for experiences wide mood swings: from periods of depression to periods of agitation and high energy.**

Frequently such mood swings will not seem connected to any actual causes.

➤ **The person you are caring for has withdrawn from others and refuses to see even good friends.**

Withdrawing from and not wanting to see others is common among depressed people.

Changing depressed feelings takes time. It usually takes at least several sessions with a counselor or therapist before a person begins to feel better. It also takes time for medicines to work, and the doctor may need to adjust the doses before the medicines are helpful.

Here is an example of what you might say when calling for professional help:

"I am Juan Alveraz, Ricardo Gonzalez's caregiver. Ricardo is a patient of Dr. Walker. He has been very discouraged since his disease has gotten worse. He is sad all of the time, refuses to talk to others, and has even stopped eating. What should I do?"

3. *WHAT YOU CAN DO TO HELP*

> ### HERE ARE THREE STEPS YOU CAN TAKE:
>
> Take care of your own emotional needs
>
> Talk about the depression
>
> Prevent or decrease depression

Take care of your own emotional needs

If you spend time on a regular basis with a person who is discouraged or depressed, it is important that you take care of your own emotional needs. Caregiving can be stressful in itself, but when the person you care for is depressed, keeping your own spirits up can be a challenge. *To do your best in this difficult role, you need to find ways to stay emotionally well yourself.* Here are some suggestions you can try:

➤ **Understand that it is not your fault that the person you are caring for is depressed.**

You should realize that you are not responsible for the other person's depression. Depression can be caused by many things, including biological changes and changes in his or her life. Sometimes, especially if the depression is severe, only professionals can help. *You should not feel guilty if, in spite of your best efforts, the person you are caring for becomes or stays depressed.*

➤ Schedule positive experiences for yourself.

To prevent becoming depressed yourself, keep doing the things outside of caregiving that make you feel good. Do not become so involved in your caregiving responsibilities that you neglect your own emotional health. Begin taking care of yourself early, and do not feel guilty about it. *Remember, if you become depressed yourself, you will not be able to provide care and support.* See the chapter "Creating and Maintaining Positive Experiences" (Chapter 19).

➤ Get the companionship you need.

Remember that you need companionship. *Being with others is as important for you as it is for the person you are caring for.* Continue to make time to be with people you like and enjoy. If you feel yourself becoming depressed, seek out other people. Some people find it helpful to talk to others about their problems. Other people find it more helpful to talk about things that have nothing to do with their problems.

➤ Get professional help for yourself, if necessary.

This can be an important part of taking care of yourself. To determine if you need professional help, read the section "When to Get Professional Help" on pp 196–198. The signs and symptoms of depression apply to you as well as to the person you are caring for.

Talk about the depression

➤ Acknowledge that the person is discouraged.

Never ignore the feelings of the person you are caring for. Sometimes people try to pretend that feelings of discouragement or depression do not exist, either because they do not want to deal with the feelings or because they hope that if they ignore the feelings, the depression will go away. *This is wrong!* It may be uncomfortable to acknowledge that someone you care about is upset, but ignoring the situation only makes it worse. The person you are caring for may feel that you do not care.

You can be of most help early—before feelings of discouragement or depression become severe. If you ignore the early signs of depression, the depression is more likely to get out of control. It is also more likely to seriously affect the quality of life of the person you are caring for and to require professional help.

> ## Agree with correct thinking.

You should make clear that you accept and agree with the thoughts that are "correct." You can also point out, in a supportive way, the "incorrect" thoughts. For example, the person you are caring for may say "I'm a total failure." *You* know that his or her whole life has not been a complete failure. You might respond to such a remark by saying, "Maybe you have failed at *some* things, but just think of all the things you have accomplished." You should then go on to talk about several of them. See the section "Techniques for Controlling Negative Thoughts" on pp 204–209 for more ideas.

> ## Encourage talking with people who have faced similar experiences.

Support groups consist of persons with similar backgrounds, experiences, and problems. It is within such groups that many people with HIV/AIDS feel truly accepted and understood. Group members share experiences that other group members can understand. Solutions to problems are discussed, and suggestions for coping are shared. All this takes place in an atmosphere of loving, caring, and support. As a caregiver, you should encourage the person you are caring for to join such support groups. Support groups for the caregivers themselves have also been formed. You can ask a social worker or nurse to refer you to any of the several support groups for persons with HIV/AIDS—or you can contact the AIDS National Interfaith Network for a referral (for more information, see Appendix A on p 307).

Prevent or decrease depression

Although the following techniques for decreasing and preventing depression work for most people, they will be helpful only if the person you are caring for cooperates. Much of the work here has to come from the person with HIV/AIDS. Both you and the person you are caring for should read the suggestions carefully and discuss them together. *Your primary role is to be a team member* by helping him or her learn these strategies and by encouraging their use.

> ## Encourage participating in pleasant, involving experiences.

Enjoyable activities can be divided into three categories: (1) activities with other people, (2) activities that give a sense of accomplishment, and (3) activities that make the person feel good. See the home care plan "Creating and Maintaining Positive Experiences" (Chapter 19) as part of your effort to help the person you are caring for combat depression. For example, being with other people is an excellent way to take attention away from negative thoughts and feelings. It provides opportunities to give and to receive help, to share experiences and perspectives, and to get help in dealing with problems. Most important, other people can express caring and love for the person with HIV/AIDS. Knowing that others care and are available to help will give the person you are caring for strength and confidence when facing an uncertain future.

Ask the person you are caring for to help you make a list of people he or she would like to spend time with. When making this list, use the following categories:

1. People who are sympathetic and understanding

2. People who give good advice and who can help solve problems

3. People who are able to help the person with HIV/AIDS turn his or her attention away from problems and toward pleasant experiences

➤ Set reasonable goals

Many people have a tendency to set goals that are too high. When they do not reach their goals, they become disheartened and sometimes give up. A person who has a progressive disease such as AIDS needs to set goals that are realistic and achievable. He or she should make plans on a daily basis and focus on short-term goals. This will allow the person to have the satisfaction of accomplishing what he sets out to do. Help the person you are caring for to realize that it is far better to set a smaller goal that can be reached than it is to set a loftier goal that is perhaps more exciting but harder to achieve. Unachieved goals can create a sense of failure. Help him or her recognize that the goals should match his or her energy level, degree of wellness, and capabilities.

➤ Point out negative thinking.

When you notice the person you are caring for expressing negative thoughts, *gently* point this out to him or her. This will help him or her to manage discouragement early, before it becomes severe. Try using a code word or phrase that the two of you agree on ahead of time to point out negative thinking. Do this early, to prevent depression from setting in.

➤ Support efforts to control repetitive negative thoughts.

When the person you are caring for lets you know that he or she is having negative thoughts and needs help to break the cycle, be available to talk about something pleasant or to do something positive with him or her. See the section "Techniques for Controlling Negative Thoughts" on pp 204–209.

> ➤ **Encourage discussing the depression with a mental health professional.**

If depression seems to be growing worse, review the section "When To Get Professional Help" on pp 196–198. Do not postpone taking action.

 ## 4. POSSIBLE OBSTACLES TO CAREGIVING

Here are some common attitudes, fears, and misconceptions that may prevent you from carrying out your plan.

"I don't want your help. Leave me alone."

Response: Explain that he or she will not feel better if you do not work together. He or she must participate if the plan is going to work, and you must be allowed to participate, too. Explain that you will not do anything without his or her permission. Have the person with HIV/AIDS read this chapter and discuss it with him or her. Agree on what you will try first. Start small—with something that is easy to do—and then think about the results.

"Of course I'm depressed: My problems are real! It's perfectly normal to be depressed in my situation."

Response: Agree that the problems are real and that having some negative feelings is normal. But suggest that he or she may become trapped in depression and that this can interfere with dealing with the problems. Explain that he or she should try to keep a balance between positive and negative thoughts. Agree that although the problems are real, the good things in life are also real and should get equal attention.

"Nothing will help, so there's no use trying."

Response: Continue to urge him or her to give it a try! Remind the person that there is nothing to lose and a good deal to gain. Encourage him or her to start with the things that are easiest to do, then discuss together whether the ideas were helpful. If the person you are caring for is so depressed that he or she cannot even try to feel better, then professional help is needed.

"I feel like I'm not helping."

Response: It is easy to get discouraged when you do not know how to help or what to do. Use this book for ideas on how you can help, and remember that being available to listen and to give support *is* a help to the person with HIV/AIDS. You do not always have to be actually "doing things" to be supportive.

Think of other obstacles

Identify additional roadblocks that could keep you from following the recommendations in this home care plan:

- Will the person I am caring for cooperate?
- Will other people help?
- How can I explain my needs to others?
- Do I have the time and energy to carry out this plan?

You need to develop plans for getting around these roadblocks. Use the four COPE ideas (*C*reativity, *O*ptimism, *P*lanning, and *E*xpert information) in developing your plans. See pp 4–8 for a discussion of how to use the four COPE ideas in overcoming your obstacles.

5. CARRYING OUT AND ADJUSTING YOUR PLAN

Carrying out your plan

➤ **Discuss this plan with the person you are helping.**

You should agree on what you will do together to manage discouragement and depression. It is important to work as a team when dealing with problems. Sometimes the support and the feeling of being a team is itself helpful.

➤ **Use the techniques suggested in this chapter early.**

Look for beginning signs of increasing discouragement or depression, and put your plan into action. Do not wait until depressed feelings are severe. The techniques discussed in this plan have helped many depressed persons. In fact, they are often a part of professional treatment. As a caregiver, you can help most if you act early.

➤ **Plan in advance what you will do to help the person you are caring for to face discouragement.**

If you know in advance what causes the person with HIV/AIDS to become discouraged, make plans for what you both will do to prevent these feelings.

➤ **Talk regularly with the person about his or her feelings.**

Although it may be difficult for you at first, let the person you are caring for know that you accept negative feelings as a reasonable response to the situation. If you are comfortable talking about feelings, the person you are caring for will feel that you care and will be more likely to let you know early on if he or she is experiencing symptoms of depression.

➤ **Persist.**

Even if the person with HIV/AIDS continues to feel depressed, do not give up. Without even realizing it, you are probably preventing depression from getting worse. Keep working cooperatively with the person you are caring for. If you are working together, it is more likely that you will succeed.

Checking on results

Continue to watch for signs that professional help is needed. Pay attention to which reconmmendations are working, and keep a "diary" of your progress.

What to do if your plan does not work

1. Review this chapter.

2. If you find that you've skipped something, try it now.

3. If you find that you've done all that you can, call the doctor for further guidance.

Ask yourself if you are expecting change too fast. It usually takes time to manage emotional problems. Look for small improvements at first. Remember, your efforts may be successful even if they merely keep negative feelings from becoming more severe.

However, if the techniques discussed in this chapter do not seem to be helping at all and the person you are caring for has been feeling depressed for several weeks, he or she should seek professional help.

 TECHNIQUES FOR CONTROLLING NEGATIVE THOUGHTS

Thought stopping

One of the most difficult things about depression is that it is so easy to get stuck in a cycle of negative thinking. Gradually you may find that depressing thoughts are merely going around and around in your head. It may seem like you cannot stop them. But you can!

The thought-stopping techniques help you to "snap out of it" as soon as that whirlpool of negative thoughts first starts. The trick is to use these techniques when you *first* notice yourself having negative thoughts:

> ## FIVE TECHNIQUES FOR CONTROLLING NEGATIVE THOUGHTS:
>
> 1. Thought stopping—to control *repetitive* negative thinking
>
> 2. Arranging a time and place for negative thinking—to *limit* negative thoughts
>
> 3. Distraction—to take *attention away from* negative thoughts
>
> 4. Arguing against negative thoughts—to show yourself how unreasonable your negative thoughts are
>
> 5. Problem solving—to solve the day-to-day problems that are *causing* negative thoughts

➤ Yell "STOP" loudly in your mind.

When you yell "STOP" in your mind, pretend it is very loud. You should pretend you are "waking yourself up"—to make yourself aware that you are in danger of getting stuck in negative thoughts. Until you become used to "shouting" in your mind, you might begin by going to an isolated place by yourself and actually shouting "STOP" out loud. Practice it this way until you can do it in your mind alone.

➤ Visualize a big red STOP sign.

Try to see it clearly. Think of what a STOP sign looks like. Make sure you see it as a red sign. First, practice seeing it in your mind so that you can bring it to mind easily. Thereafter, whenever you catch yourself starting negative thoughts, think of this image and stop yourself. Then immediately turn your thoughts to something else.

➤ Splash some water on your face.

Splashing water on your face is another way to "wake yourself up" from negative thinking. Pay attention to how the water makes you feel and stop your negative thoughts.

➤ Get up and move to a new spot.

Getting up and moving to a new spot will give you a change of scenery. After you move to the new spot, use the new surroundings to help you think about other things—for example, think about the things that you *see*.

When you are feeling negative, you may consider these techniques to be "silly" and may think to yourself "How could anything so simple possibly work?" Actually, research has demonstrated that they *can* work. Give them a try! *You have to fight the negative thoughts. Maybe trying several of these together will work for you.*

Arranging a time and a place for negative thinking

This technique allows you to think occasionally about negative things, but puts *you* in control of when and where you do this thinking.

➤ **Find a negative thinking "place."**

This can be a particular room, a special chair, or maybe even by a certain window. Make this the *only* place you let yourself have negative thoughts. Your negative thinking space can be any place you choose. Do not, however, make it your bed or the place where you eat. These need to be "safe zones."

➤ **Schedule a time each day for thinking negative thoughts.**

You might not be able to control all negative thinking, especially in the beginning. Scheduling a specific time to have negative thoughts helps you to take control of them.

Do not make this time around mealtimes, just before you go to sleep, or just before you expect to see people. These should be relaxing times. Also, allow this time to last for no longer than 15 minutes. At the end of 15 minutes, stop. You can "continue" these thoughts the following day.

This exercise give you control of when and where you think negative thoughts.

Distraction

You cannot think of two things at once. When you find yourself starting to think negative thoughts, get your mind involved in another thought "activity" that "pushes out" or replaces the negative thinking. These exercises are also helpful when you are feeling anxious and need help falling asleep. Try one of the following ideas:

➤ **Take a "vacation" in your mind.**

Close your eyes and think about your favorite spot or event—for example, a party. Spend a couple minutes there on a mental vacation. Relax and enjoy it.

Really try to work your imagination. Think about as many details as possible.

What does it feel like? Is there a warm breeze? Imagine how it will feel on your skin.

What does it look like? Is the sky clear and blue? Or are you in a room? Imagine what the room looks like. Try to see it as completely as you can.

What does it smell like? Is there a salty smell of the ocean? Maybe you smell the fragrances of a garden or a big dinner. Make it as clear as you can.

Are you drinking a nice cool drink? What does it taste like? Feel it in your mouth. Taste it.

➤ **Mental "time travel" into the future.**

Think of something that you are looking forward to. Imagine that it is happening. Think of how nice it is to be there.

➤ **Practice relaxation.**

Use the relaxation exercise outlined in the home care plan "Coping with Anxiety" (Chapter 18). Being relaxed helps you to think about pleasant things.

➤ **Do something you enjoy.**

Get yourself involved in an activity you enjoy. Filling your mind with positive thoughts or activities will help "crowd out" the negative thoughts.

Arguing against negative thoughts

This technique will help you see both sides of the picture. Things are not usually as bad as they first seem when you are depressed. One way to see the other side is to actively argue against the negative view.

You can fight your negative thoughts. Challenge their accuracy. Every situation has at least two sides to it. When you are depressed, you probably only see the bad side; ordinarily you would try to look at both sides. Play the "part" of someone who is arguing with you to get you to see the bright side of the situation. Practice having a debate with yourself, and try to ensure that the positive side "wins."

➤ **Ask yourself if the negative thought is actually true.**

Make yourself be clear about what evidence supports it.

➤ **Now take the other side.**

Think of every reason why your thoughts may be exaggerated or not true, and make a strong argument for the "positive" side.

Do not give up easily. Really argue as if you were arguing with someone else. When you are arguing against your negative thoughts, try to be as complete as possible. You may want to write down answers to the following questions:

What is the evidence against my negative thoughts?

Are there any "facts" in my thinking that are not backed up by truth?

Is my argument an example of "black and white" thinking? Are there shades of gray that I'm ignoring?

Is the negative side taking things out of focus? Am I looking at the whole picture or just one small part of it?

Am I trying to predict the future, when I know that I can't?

Try to punch as many holes in the "negative side" of your argument as you can. Do not accept any illogical thinking.

Problem Solving: Solving the day-to-day problems that are causing negative thoughts

Use a problem-solving approach to overcome some of the day-to-day problems that are contributing to your feelings of depression, such as finding enough time to do housework, problems with family members, and so on.

The home care plan "Solving Problems Using the *Home Care Guide for HIV/AIDS*" (Chapter 1) explains in greater detail how to use four problem-solving steps to deal with problems that are not included in this book. The four steps are as follows:

1. Be **creative** in dealing with obstacles. Try seeing the problem from someone else's perspective, asking other people for ideas, and rethinking your expectations.

2. Be both **optimistic** and realistic.

3. Develop an orderly **plan**. Review the facts, set reasonable goals, and choose strategies that are the best balance between risk and benefit.

4. Make effective use of **expert information**—the kind of information that is in the *Home Care Guide for HIV/AIDS*.

You can remember these four key approaches by thinking of the word COPE (which means to succeed in solving problems):

C for Creativity

O for Optimism

P for Planning

E for Expert information

Research has shown that people who use the four COPE techniques are better problem solvers. Research has also shown that people who use the four COPE techniques experience less stress when dealing with problems.

Coping with Anxiety

Overview of the Home Care Plan for
Anxiety

1. **UNDERSTANDING THE PROBLEM**

Symptoms of anxiety

How persons with HIV/AIDS may experience prolonged anxiety

Causes of anxiety for persons with HIV/AIDS

Your goals

2. **WHEN TO GET PROFESSIONAL HELP**

Symptoms that indicate the need for professional help

What to say when you call

3. **WHAT YOU CAN DO TO HELP**

Find out what is causing the anxiety

Encourage conversation about concerns and fears

Encourage the use of relaxation techniques

Encourage the person you are caring for to engage in pleasant, distracting activities

4. **POSSIBLE OBSTACLES TO CAREGIVING**

5. **CARRYING OUT AND ADJUSTING YOUR PLAN**

Carrying out your plan

Checking on results

What to do if your plan does not work

Topics that have an arrow (➤) in front of them are actions you can take or symptoms you can look for.

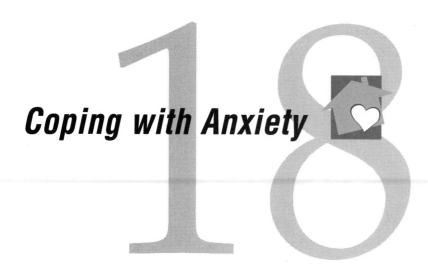

Coping with Anxiety

The person you are caring for is the one who will use the techniques and information in this home care plan to help him or her face anxiety. You, the caregiver, may also use the techniques discussed in this chapter, if you find that you are anxious. Work together as a team to get the most out of this home care plan.

1. UNDERSTANDING THE PROBLEM

Everyone experiences anxiety from time to time. Anxiety may be a feeling as mild as "nervousness" or "tension," or it may be described as a more intense feeling, such as "fear" or "panic." Anxiety may be described as a sense of dread that "something bad is going to happen" or as "losing control." Often, it is accompanied by physical symptoms, such as sweaty palms, an "upset stomach," trembling, or difficulty breathing.

In most people, anxiety comes and goes fairly quickly. However, when anxiety is prolonged or severe, it can interfere with quality of life.

People with HIV/AIDS are especially likely to experience prolonged anxiety. They have many valid reasons to be fearful and anxious.

> ➤ The information in this home care plan fits most situations, but yours may be different.
>
> ➤ If the doctor or nurse tells you to do something else, follow what he or she says.
>
> ➤ See the section "When To Get Professional Help" on p 215.

Common causes of anxiety in people with HIV/AIDS include

1. Worries about medical procedures

2. Fear of being a burden to family and friends

3. Fear of pain and discomfort

4. Side effects of HIV/AIDS treatment medicines

5. Fear of becoming sicker

6. Fear of death

Anxiety may also make other symptoms more intense. For example, a person who is in pain usually reports that pain is more severe when he or she is anxious.

Controlling anxiety is primarily in the hands of the person with HIV/AIDS. However, one of the difficulties of anxiety is that it is not always easy to recognize: The person experiencing the anxiety may believe that he or she is merely "worried." Sometimes it is easier for family and friends to recognize anxiety than it is for the person who is experiencing it. Helping the person with HIV/AIDS to recognize his or her anxiety and encouraging him or her to talk about fears and concerns will therefore help control the anxiety and keep it from becoming severe. *You should work with the person you are caring for as a team to control and reduce the anxiety.* Also, remember that family and friends caring for a person with HIV/AIDS may likewise experience anxiety caused by dealing with the illness. Sometimes the anxiety of the person with HIV/AIDS makes the caregivers anxious themselves. Other times, poor communication between the person who is ill and family and friends is the source of anxiety. It is important for you to take care of your own emotional needs, too. Therefore, you should read this chapter both to help the person you are caring for and also to help yourself.

Because anxiety is a normal response to new or stressful situations, do not expect to eliminate all anxiety. What you and the person with HIV/AIDS can do together is prevent anxiety from becoming so severe that it interferes with his or her quality of life.

YOUR GOALS

Know when to call for professional help

Find out what is causing the anxiety

Encourage conversation about concerns and fears

Encourage the use of relaxation techniques

Encourage the person you are caring for to engage in pleasant, distracting activities

---

2. WHEN TO GET PROFESSIONAL HELP

Some people are hesitant to ask for help with emotional problems because they do not want to appear "crazy." They should understand that having emotional problems during a major illness is perfectly normal—and that getting help for these problems is normal, too.

When seeking professional help, it is best to start with the doctor treating the disease, who is familiar with the person you are caring for and with the stage of his or her illness. Ask for an evaluation of the causes of the anxiety as well as for treatment recommendations.

If the anxiety is severe, the health care professional may use special techniques such as anti-anxiety medicines or stress management techniques.

You may also ask for a referral to a mental health professional. Mental health professionals (psychologists, psychiatrists, and social workers) are experienced in helping people with emotional problems. Many mental health professionals have experience treating people with HIV/AIDS and the depression that is brought on by the stress of the illness. Signs that the person you are caring for requires professional help include the following:

➤ **Anxiety that is causing the person you are caring for to seriously consider stopping treatments and medications, skipping treatments, or avoiding visits to the doctor.**

➤ **The person you are caring for is currently experiencing anxiety *and has had a history of severe anxiety requiring professional help or therapy in the past*.**

➤ **Anxiety that is interfering with ordinary daily acitivities and that is significantly affecting the quality of life of the person you are caring for.**

Anxiety that lasts for several days in a row can interfere with sleep and accomplishing normal everyday tasks such as eating or bathing.

Here is an example of what you might say when calling for professional help:

"I am John Brown, Pete Stone's caregiver. I am very concerned because Pete is complaining about symptoms of shakiness; fears that come on at night and make it difficult for him to sleep; and feelings of panic over difficulty breathing. Pete is just anxious all of the time about one thing or another. What should I do?"

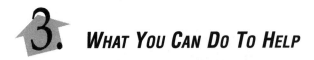

WHAT YOU CAN DO TO HELP

> **HERE ARE FOUR STEPS YOU CAN TAKE:**
>
> Find out what is causing the fear and anxiety
>
> Encourage conversation about concerns and fears
>
> Encourage the use of relaxation techniques
>
> Encourage the person you are caring for to engage in pleasant, distracting activities

Find out what is causing the fear and anxiety

➤ **Ask questions that help to point to the sources of anxiety.**

Finding out what thoughts are causing the anxiety or fear is the key to controlling them. Anxiety has two parts: thoughts and feelings. Disturbing thoughts lead to feelings of nervousness or anxiety. Feelings of nervousness, in turn, can lead to more disturbing thoughts. To help the person you are caring for stop this cycle, you first need to find out what thoughts are causing the anxiety. Ask the person *why* those thoughts are causing anxiety.

Ask the person you are caring for specific questions about what he or she believes is the source of anxiety. Questions to ask may include the following:

Is he or she anxious about medical treatments? If so, why? Ask the person to explain what *exactly* it is about the medical treatments that is causing anxiety.

Are the fears connected with feeling so sick?

Does he or she sense that the disease is getting out of control?

Are the fears related to death? Does the person believe that he or she is going to die soon?

Is the person afraid that he or she will be unable to cope with the disease and required treatment?

Is the person anxious about receiving medical information? If so, exactly what kind of news is he or she afraid of learning? For example, is it news that his or her CD4 counts are very low and that the disease is rapidly advancing? Or is it news that an AIDS-related cancer or some other complication has developed?

It is important to be tactful and sensitive when asking these types of questions. Just talking about such things may upset the person you are caring for even further. Being tactful and showing that you care, on the other hand, may help comfort the person.

Encourage conversation about concerns and fears

➤ **Encourage the person you are caring for to join a support group for persons with HIV/AIDS.**

Support groups are self-help groups that enable people with similar problems to meet, share concerns, and support each other emotionally. Hearing about how someone else overcame or is dealing with a difficult experience, especially if the experience is similar, can help provide solutions to anxiety. It may even be reassuring to the person you are caring for just to feel that he or she "is not alone." You can ask a health care professional to refer you to any of the several support groups that now exist for persons with HIV/AIDS—or you can contact the AIDS National Interfaith Network for a referral **(for more information, see Appendix A on p 307).**

Encourage the use of relaxation techniques

Many persons with HIV/AIDS have found relaxation techniques helpful. These techniques can be used anytime—even for short periods of time. Try the following relaxation exercise yourself to see how it feels and works for you. This will help you to support the person with HIV/AIDS in using relaxation techniques.

Relaxation techniques should be practiced at least once a day but not within an hour after a meal because the digestion process may interfere with the ability to relax certain muscles.

Both you and the person you are caring for should read this exercise. He or she may want you to help. If so, you can read these instructions out loud while he or she tries the technique. *This exercise should be performed only when you are not feeling rushed.*

1. Sit quietly in a comfortable position (such as an easy chair or sofa).

2. Close your eyes.

3. Deeply relax your muscles, beginning with the face and going throughout the entire body (shoulders, chest, arms, hands, stomach, legs) and ending with the feet. Allow the tension to "flow out through your feet."

4. Now turn your attention to your head and relax your head even further by thinking "I'm going to let all the tension flow out of my head. I'm letting go of the tension and I'm letting warm feelings of relaxation smooth out the muscles in my head and face. I'm becoming more relaxed."

5. Repeat this last step for different parts of your body: your shoulders, arms, hands, chest, abdomen, legs, and feet. Do this

slowly—spend enough time to feel more relaxed before going on to the next part of the body.

6. Once the body feels very relaxed, turn your attention to your breathing. Become aware of how rhythmic and deep your breathing has become. Breathe slowly and deeply. Breathe through your nose. As you breathe out, say the word "Calm" silently to yourself. Slowly take a breath in. Now slowly let it out and silently say "Calm" to yourself. Repeat this with every breath. It helps you to relax more if you concentrate on just this one word "Calm." Continue breathing deeply, becoming more and more relaxed.

7. Continue this exercise for 10 to 15 minutes more. You should remain relaxed, breathing slowly. At the end of the exercise, open your eyes gradually to become adjusted to the light in the room, and sit quietly for a few minutes.

When the exercise is over, ask yourself how relaxed you became and if there were any problems in doing it. A common problem is drifting and distracting thoughts. If a distracting thought occurs, let it pass. Let it fly away, like a bird. Don't fight it. Don't give up because of distracting thoughts. Your relaxation technique is a process, and distracting thoughts will always occur. Just push them away gently and continue. Concentrate more on the word "Calm." Let the thought drift by and repeat "Calm" over and over again as your breathing gets more slow and deep—as you relax more and more. Remind yourself to "let relaxation happen at its own pace," and don't allow yourself to become impatient or anxious about being unable to relax "fast enough."

After you have become skilled at this exercise, you will find that it is easy to apply as soon as you are getting tense. For example, if you feel tense while waiting to see the doctor or are waiting for some test results, you can easily close your eyes for a few minutes and use this exercise to relax and feel calm.

To get the most benefit from this technique:

- Perform this exercise at least once a day. In the beginning it may help to have someone else give you the instructions. You may also record these instructions on an inexpensive tape recorder and play them when you are relaxing.

- When you practice this exercise, choose a time when you will not be disturbed. Tell the other people in your household what you are doing and ask them to be as quiet as possible while you are doing this exercise.

- Learn this relaxation technique early, to prevent anxiety from becoming severe.

Encourage the person you are caring for to engage in pleasant, distracting activities

➤ **Encourage the person you are caring for to choose activities that are fun, satisfying, and energizing**

Engaging in activities that are pleasant and relaxing can take his or her mind off of problems and worries. See the home care plan "Creating and Maintaining Positive Experiences" (Chapter 19) for ideas on planning enjoyable activities.

➤ **Encourage the person you are caring for to spend time with friends and family members who care.**

Knowing that other people care and are available can help the person you are caring for to more confidently face anxiety-provoking experiences. It can also give family and friends the opportunity to express caring and love.

The home care plan "Getting Companionship and Support" (Chapter 20) guides you in developing plans for increasing the amount of support the person with HIV/AIDS receives from other people.

4. POSSIBLE OBSTACLES TO CAREGIVING

Here are some common attitudes and misconceptions that may prevent you from carrying out your plan:

"My problems are real: That's why I worry about them."

Response: Agree that the problems are real and that worrying about them is normal and understandable. However, remind him or her that anxiety that is not managed correctly may become severe. Point out that research has shown that severe anxiety interferes with the ability to solve problems. If you notice that the anxiety has already become severe, encourage the person you are caring for to seek professional help.

"I can't stop the thoughts that make me scared. They keep coming back and racing around my head."

Response: Encourage him or her to try various techniques for stopping negative thoughts. Some techniques are discussed in the home care plan "Coping with Depression" (Chapter 17) on pp 204–209. You might also have him or her practice the relaxation exercise discussed earlier in this chapter. These are helpful in stopping repetitive unpleasant thoughts.

"I'm feeling stressed out myself. I've been under stress for so long from taking care of someone who is seriously ill that I feel anxious all the time. This makes it very hard for me to help other people with their emotional problems.

Response: Spending a great deal of time with someone who has long-standing anxiety can be very stressful and can cause you to become anxious yourself. You need to take time for yourself to deal with your own stress. Use the strategies discussed in this chapter for *yourself*: Talk with others who have gone through a similar experience (for example, other people who have cared for a seriously ill family member) or attend a support group; continue to engage in satisfying, pleasant activities; practice relaxation techniques; and spend time with people who care. If you think that you might need professional help, read the section "When to Get Professional Help" on p 215. The signs and symptoms of severe anxiety apply to you as well as to the person you are caring for. Also, see the home care plans "Creating and Maintaining Positive Experiences" (Chapter 19), "Getting Companionship and Support" (Chapter 20), and "Coping with Depression" (Chapter 17) for further ideas on how to take care of your own needs. You should also involve as many people as possible in carrying out this home care plan. Extra support will help both you and the person with HIV/AIDS.

Think of other obstacles

Identify additional roadblocks that could keep you from following the recommendations in this home care plan:

- Will the person I am caring for cooperate?

- Will other people help?

- How can I explain my needs to others?

- Do I have the time and energy to carry out this plan?

You need to develop plans for getting around these roadblocks. Use the four COPE ideas (*C*reativity, *O*ptimism, *P*lanning, and *E*xpert information) in developing your plans. See pp 4–8 for a discussion of how to use the four COPE ideas in overcoming your obstacles.

 ## CARRYING OUT AND ADJUSTING YOUR PLAN

Carrying out your plan

➤ **Talk this plan over with the person you are caring for.**

Remember that you are a team. You should agree together on what you will try to manage anxiety.

➤ **Make plans in advance for managing anxiety.**

If you know when anxiety is most likely to occur, you can make plans in advance for preventing or minimizing these feelings.

Checking on results

➤ **Continue to watch for signs that professional help is needed.**

➤ **Talk regularly about emotional feelings, just as you do about physical feelings.**

Keep a daily log of anxiety levels. Ask the person you are caring for to rate his or her anxiety on a scale of 0 to 10, with 0 being no anxiety and 10 being the worst anxiety ever experienced. Make a note about which activities or events caused anxiety and which ones were relaxing. Pay attention to which recommendations in this home care plan are working. This will help you prevent further anxiety and keep it from becoming serious.

What to do if your plan does not work

1. Review this chapter.

2. If you find that you've skipped something, try it now.

3. If you find that you've done all that you can, call the doctor for further guidance.

Ask yourself if you are expecting change too fast. It usually takes time to manage emotional problems. Look for small improvement at first. Remember, your efforts are successful even if they merely keep anxiety from becoming more severe.

However, if the techniques discussed in this chapter do not seem to be helping at all and the person you are caring for has been feeling anxious for several weeks, he or she should seek professional help.

19

Creating and Maintaining Positive Experiences

Overview of the Home Care Plan for
Creating and Maintaining Positive Experiences

 1. **UNDERSTANDING THE PROBLEM**

> Why positive experiences are important during an illness
>
> Creating positive experiences for yourself, too

2. **WHEN TO GET PROFESSIONAL HELP**

> Symptoms that indicate the need for professional help
>
> What to say when you call

3. **WHAT YOU CAN DO TO HELP**

> Encourage positive, enjoyable activities
>
> Help the person you are caring for to pay attention to positive experiences
>
> Plan activities in which the person you are caring for can participate
>
> Examples of how activities done in the past can be done now changed

 4. **POSSIBLE OBSTACLES TO CAREGIVING**

5. **CARRYING OUT AND ADJUSTING YOUR PLAN**

> Carrying out your plan
>
> Checking on results
>
> What to do if your plan does not work

Topics that have an arrow (➤) in front of them are actions you can take or symptoms you can look for.

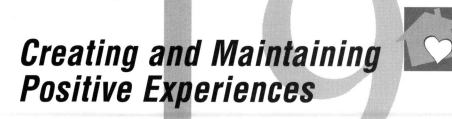

Creating and Maintaining Positive Experiences

1. UNDERSTANDING THE PROBLEM

People with HIV/AIDS, like so many others who face chronic illnesses, tend to focus their attention only on the illness and the problems it creates. As a result, they lose interest in others and stop participating in activities that they used to enjoy. They may give up favorite pastimes or hobbies and may isolate themselves from others. (For more on the latter problem, see the home care plan "Getting Companionship and Support," Chapter 20). By doing this, they can get stuck in the role of the "sick person," and their whole life may begin to revolve around just that.

Pleasant, satisfying experiences help people to cope with the stresses and difficulties of ill health. Having fun helps people feel better physically and emotionally. When a person regularly does things that are enjoyable, he or she will keep a positive outlook on life and be less likely to become discouraged during a difficult illness such as HIV/AIDS.

> ➤ The information in this home care plan fits most situations, but yours may be different.
>
> ➤ If the doctor or nurse tells you to do something else, follow what he or she says.
>
> ➤ See the section "When To Get Professional Help" on pp 196–198.

The purpose of this chapter is to help the person with HIV/AIDS to consider things in his or her life other than the illness and problems related to it. This will help keep negativity, anxiety, and depression from setting in.

Caregivers of persons with HIV/AIDS can also become preoccupied with problems. Caregivers, too, need to remember to participate in enjoyable activities, to maintain a positive outlook on life. If you think only about the needs and problems of the person with HIV/AIDS, you are likely to become upset and discouraged. For this reason, you should use this home care plan for yourself as well as for the person you are caring for.

YOUR GOALS

Know when to get professional help

Encourage positive, enjoyable activities

Help the person you are caring for to pay attention to positive experiences

Plan activities in which the person with HIV/AIDS can participate

---

2. WHEN TO GET PROFESSIONAL HELP

Sometimes, despite your best efforts to involve the person you are caring for in positive experiences, he or she will remain depressed. If depression is severe or continues for more than 2 weeks, professional help is needed. For a list of specific signs that professional help is needed, refer to pp 196–198, the section "When to Get Professional Help" in the home care plan "Coping with Depression" (Chapter 17).

3. WHAT YOU CAN DO TO HELP

HERE ARE FOUR STEPS YOU CAN TAKE:

Encourage positive, enjoyable activities

Pay attention to positive experiences

Plan activities in which the person with HIV/AIDS can participate

Change favorite activities of the past to fit the present situation

---

Encourage positive, enjoyable activities

There are three types of positive experiences that are not only enjoyable but also important for maintaining good quality of life. These can help to prevent discouragement or depression.

> **Enjoyable activities with other people.**

Examples include:

Talking with a friend about mutual interests

Shopping with a friend

Going to the beach with friends

Calling a friend on the phone

Going to a party given by friends

Playing cards with friends

Going to church

Singing in a choir

Attending a support group

Attending a play, movie, or concert with friends

You will know that the person you are caring for is noticing pleasant things that happened with others when you hear comments such as: "Jerry said I looked good today;" "Martha went out of her way to get my medicine;" "Mary and I had a good talk;" or "Bill and I talked about the old days."

> **Activities that give a sense of accomplishment and pride.**

Examples include:

Cooking a meal or part of a meal

Arranging a photo album

Repairing a broken lamp

Starting a new hobby

Beginning an exercise program

Solving a crossword puzzle

Writing a letter, a poem, or a song

Volunteer work

Playing a musical instrument

Restoring old furniture

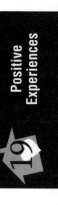

Positive Experiences

Cleaning the house

Keeping a journal

Supporting a friend who is in need

You will know that the person you are caring for is experiencing a sense of accomplishment when you hear comments such as: "I beat Charlie at chess;" "I finished knitting the arm to the sweater;" "I cleaned out my bureau drawers;" "I balanced the checkbook;" "I finished potting the flowers;" "I walked even farther today than I did yesterday."

➤ **Activities that make the person feel good.**

Examples include:

Watching a favorite TV program

Watching a funny movie

Taking a ride in the country

Listening to a favorite kind of music

Walking along the seashore or in the park

Hugging a loved one

Eating a favorite food

Saying a prayer

Playing with a pet

Going to a religious service

Reading a good book or favorite magazine

You will know that the person you are caring for is benefitting from these activities when you hear comments such as: "It was a beautiful day for a walk in the countryside;" "I really laughed at the interview on the evening news;" "I went to church;" "I ordered flowers for Ann who is in the hospital;" "I encouraged Bill who was just diagnosed with HIV."

Help the person you are caring for pay attention to positive experiences

➤ **Talk about pleasant experiences as they happen during the day.**

When a person is under stress, it is easy to notice and think only about unpleasant experiences. When this happens, it can make you and the person with HIV/AIDS depressed. Make a point of noticing and talking about all of the pleasant things *as they hap-*

pen. For example, if you are with the person you are caring for and you notice that a sales clerk is being especially courteous, you might point this out as soon as you leave the store, by saying something like "That sales clerk certainly tried to be helpful, didn't she?"

> **Set aside time each evening for you and the person you are caring for to recall the good things that happened that day.**

Think back over the day and talk with him or her about everything pleasant that happened that day. Focus on small things as well as important things.

> **Recall pleasant experiences from the past.**

Remember pleasant activities from the past and the times you had fun doing different things together. This can help to create positive feelings for both of you.

> **Make lists of pleasant experiences or activities and read them over from time to time.**

Doing so reminds the person you are caring for about the good things that have occurred and that can occur again. If you do this for a while, you will both find yourselves noticing good things as they happen and will start the day looking forward to the positive things that can happen.

Plan activities that the person you are caring for can engage in

> **Make a list of activities that have been pleasant and enjoyable in the past.**

Take your time doing this so that the list will be as complete as possible. Include activities that have been pleasant during the illness, as well as before the illness.

> **Decide which of these activities can reasonably be planned for now.**

Some activities will not require any changes. Others may have to be changed because of limitations due to the illness. Consider whether (1) the person you are caring for can do at least part of a favorite activity; and (2) whether something similar to the activity can be done.

Adjust favorite activities of the past to fit the present situation

Here are some examples of how favorite activities of the past activities can be adjusted so that the person you are caring for can do at least part of them or something similar to them now:

> *Enjoyable activities with other people:*
> All-day shopping excursion with friends *BECOMES*
>   A short trip to the store with friends
> Dinner out at a restaurant with friends BECOMES
>   Inviting friends over to your house for dessert
> Playing on a sports team BECOMES Watching baseball
>   on TV with a friend
>
> *Important activities that give a sense of accomplishment:*
> Cleaning the house BECOMES Clean one room
> Sailing BECOMES Build a model sailboat
>
> *Activities that make him or her feel good:*
> Going to the movies BECOMES Rent a video
> Going to concerts BECOMES Play records after supper

4. POSSIBLE OBSTACLES TO CAREGIVING

Here are some common attitudes and misconception that may prevent you from carrying out your plan:

"I'm so depressed and upset that no activity is pleasant anymore."

Response: No matter how depressed a person is, there are always *some* activities and thoughts that are pleasant—even if only for a short time. Start by watching for the good things that happen each day, no matter how small they may be, and to discuss them or just think them over at the end of the day. As the next step, try planning different activities until you find something that he or she responds to. It may be "slow-going" at first, but keep trying. You will often find that he or she will gradually become more and more responsive. However, if the person is so depressed that he or she does not even want to try to feel better, professional help is needed. (See the home care plan "Coping with Depression" [Chapter 17] for further suggestions on dealing with depression.)

"When you are sick a lot of things happen that you wish wouldn't happen—but you can't do anything about them."

Response: The person you are caring for may not be able to change many of the problems caused by the illness, but he or she *can* balance the negative experiences with experiences that are positive.

"I have so many problems to deal with that I can't find time for pleasant activities."

Response: Remind him or her that pleasant activities are especially important for people who are under stress. *Make time for pleasant experiences, even in the midst of problems.* Work with him or her to write a realistic schedule that includes pleasant activities.

"I feel guilty if I enjoy myself when the person I'm caring for feels sick and needs my help."

Response: Do *not* feel guilty. You should be scheduling pleasant experiences for yourself as well as for the person you are caring for. You will be a more effective caregiver if you are in good spirits and doing things you enjoy. If you are tired and worn out, you will not be able to do your best as a caregiver. *Scheduling pleasant experiences for yourself is part of being an effective caregiver.*

Think of other obstacles

Identify additional roadblocks that could keep you from following the recommendations in this home care plan:

- Will the person I am caring for cooperate?

- Will other people help?

- How can I explain my needs to others?

- Do I have the time and energy to carry out this plan?

You need to develop plans for getting around these roadblocks. Use the four COPE ideas (Creativity, Optimism, Planning, and Expert information) in developing your plans. See pp 4–8 for a discussion of how to use the four COPE ideas in overcoming your obstacles.

5. CARRYING OUT AND ADJUSTING YOUR PLAN

Carrying out your plan

➤ **Start now.**

Do not wait until the person you are caring for is depressed or feeling overwhelmed by problems. Start using this home care plan right away and then continue to use it throughout the illness. Start by noticing positive things as they happen. At the end of the day, make lists of the good things that happened, and finally, schedule pleasant activities to do each week. Scheduling pleasant activities is one of the best ways to protect against depression.

➤ **Set deadlines.**

If you do not set deadlines for engaging in pleasant activities, problems will push them aside. Therefore, you should decide,

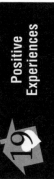

with the person you care for, when you will do each of the activities you listed.

Checking on results

Pay attention to which activities are most helpful to the person you are caring for. *Listen* to what he or she tells you, and keep notes or a "diary" on these comments. Your lists of good things that happen each day will be a record of your progress.

What to do if your plan does not work

1. Review this chapter.

2. If you find that you've skipped something, try it now.

3. If you find that you've done all that you can, call the doctor for further guidance.

Try not to become discouraged if you are not successful right away. As you get more experience, you will get better and better at planning and noticing positive experiences. Ask yourself if your goals have been reasonable, or if you have been expecting change too fast. Perhaps you have been setting goals that are too ambitious.

Ask other people to make suggestions of pleasant activities for the person you are caring for. Other caregivers may have good ideas. Social workers and nurses who work with HIV/AIDS patients often have good suggestions. Be creative, and try unusual and new ideas.

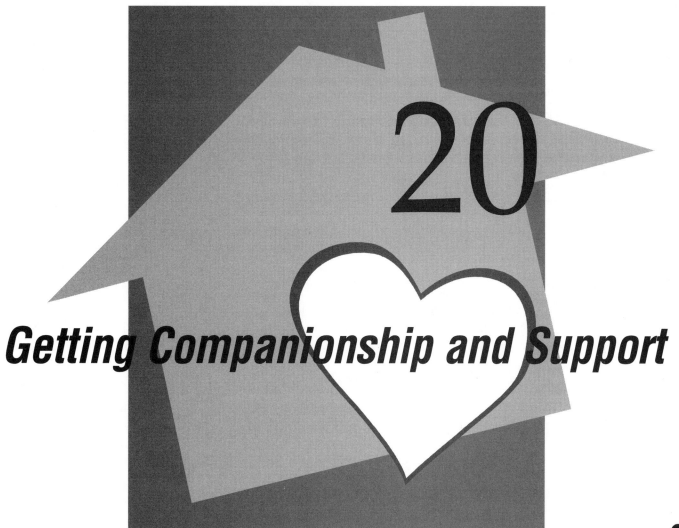

Getting Companionship and Support

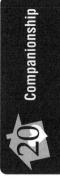

Overview of the Home Care Plan for
Getting Companionship and Support

 1. UNDERSTANDING THE PROBLEM

    Reasons for people failing to visit

    The importance of companionship

    The role of the caregiver in finding companionship for
    the person with HIV/AIDS

    Your goals

 2. WHEN TO GET PROFESSIONAL HELP

    Symptoms that indicate the need for professional help

 3. WHAT YOU CAN DO TO HELP

    Invite others to visit

    Make visits pleasant experiences

    Find other ways of getting companionship

 4. POSSIBLE OBSTACLES TO CAREGIVING

 5. CARRYING OUT AND ADJUSTING YOUR PLAN

    Checking on results

    What to do if your plan does not work

**Topics that have an arrow (➤) in front
of them are actions you can take or
symptoms you can look for.**

Getting Companionship and Support

1. UNDERSTANDING THE PROBLEM

In general, when a person is sick, loved ones and friends tend to express concern and usually offer to help. Although many people are very interested and concerned early in the illness, what often happens is that fewer and fewer people take the time and effort to visit or to call as the illness goes on. This happens for several reasons. Sometimes people who are not sick find that they are too uncomfortable around those who are, especially when the disease is a chronic illness such as HIV/AIDS.

In addition, the stigma attached to having HIV/AIDS may keep some family members and friends away. At the same time, many people with HIV/AIDS tend to withdraw from old friends and family members, especially as their illness progresses, because they do not want other people to see them when they are so ill. Sometimes persons with HIV/AIDS avoid others because they think other people will try to tell them what to do or will say things that make them feel guilty. Other times, persons with HIV/AIDS just do not have the energy to visit with others. This can make family and friends feel

> ➤ The information in this home care plan fits most situations, but yours may be different.
>
> ➤ If the doctor or nurse tells you to do something else, follow what he or she says.
>
> ➤ See the section "When To Get Professional Help" on pp 196–198.

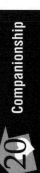

unwelcome. Unfortunately, a very important part of life is lost when the person with HIV/AIDS sees fewer and fewer people. The person loses the stimulation of thinking about other people's lives, the ability to see his or her own problems in a larger perspective, and the help and comfort that others can give. He or she also grows to feel that other people do not love or care about him or her. Losing contact with friends or loved ones in this manner can contribute significantly to depression.

It is important that you, as a caregiver, do what you can to prevent social isolation. You should invite selected people. Organize their visits so that they are helpful to the person with HIV/AIDS and rewarding for the visitors so that they will want to come again. This chapter discusses ways of getting companionship and support for the person you are caring for—and for *yourself*, too.

Your goal in carrying out this plan is to arrange for as much social contact as the person with HIV/AIDS needs and wants throughout the illness.

Remember that your own needs for companionship and support are also important. You will be a more effective caregiver if you keep up your outside interests and relationships with other people during this illness. You should use the ideas in this chapter for yourself as well. Planning time away with friends can be very helpful. It can take your thoughts away from caregiving, or it can give you a chance to tell others about your feelings and difficulties. It can also give others an opportunity to express their support to you and to make suggestions from their experiences.

YOUR GOALS

Know when to get professional help

Invite others to visit

Make visits pleasant experiences

Find other ways of getting companionship

 ## WHEN TO GET PROFESSIONAL HELP

Sometimes, even if the person you are caring is getting all the support and companionship he or she needs, depression may remain a problem. If depression is severe or continues for more than 2 weeks, professional help is needed. For a list of specific signs that professional help should be sought, refer to pp 196–198, the section "When To Get Professional Help" in the home care plan "Coping with Depression" (Chapter 17).

---

3. WHAT YOU CAN DO TO HELP

> **HERE ARE THREE STEPS YOU CAN TAKE:**
>
> Invite others to visit
>
> Make visits pleasant experiences
>
> Find other ways of getting companionship

Invite others to visit

Do not wait for visits simply to "happen," or for people to invite themselves over. Take steps yourself to ensure that people visit the person you are caring for. Develop a plan for inviting people to your home.

➤ **Make a list of the people whom you would like to have visit.**

Part of your job as a caregiver is to encourage visits. Ask the person you are caring for to help you make a list of people he or she would like to spend time with. When making this list, use the following categories:

1. People who are sympathetic and understanding

2. People who give good advice and who can help solve problems

3. People who are able to help the person with HIV/AIDS turn his or her attention away from problems and toward pleasant experiences

Consider persons who are important to him or her. Discuss with the person the types of people he or she would like to see. Consider the following: friends, people from work, close family members, a minister or other church members, people who belong to the same support group as the person with HIV/AIDS, people with same life interests, and people who are comfortable being around someone who is ill.

➤ **Discuss how you will invite others to visit.**

After you and the person you are caring for have discussed who should visit, decide who will do the inviting. If he or she feels weak or "out of sorts," you can offer to do this. Decide together how you will invite others. A telephone call is probably the easiest way to contact others, but you could write notes. It is very important that you respect the wishes of the person who is ill. Encourage him or her to have visitors, but do not force the issue.

Companionship

20

Make visits pleasant experiences

Visits are more likely to be positive experiences for everyone involved if you plan them in advance. When visits are pleasant, people are more likely to want to come back.

➤ **Find out what would make the visit most comfortable and enjoyable** *for both the person you are caring for and for the visitors.*

Discuss this with person you are caring for. Have him or her decide ahead of time how long a visit should last and what should and should not happen during that visit. Consider activities other than just conversation. Card games, working on puzzles, listening to music, or watching a favorite movie could be things all could enjoy. Have some ideas in mind for each visit, and plan them with the person who is ill before visitors come. However, others might like a short chat in which both parties do some "catching up" on events in their lives. Remind the person to avoid conversation that focuses on just the illness. Light conversation, laughing, and joking are good medicine.

➤ **Help visitors to feel welcome and at ease.**

Many people feel awkward when around a person who is ill. They may not know what to say or what questions are OK to ask. Tell visitors ahead of time about the state of illness or wellness they will find when they enter the home. Let them know what topics are OK to discuss and which, if any, the ill person is uncomfortable talking about that day. If people are prepared to see a weaker or thinner person, there is less surprise and less feelings of awkwardness.

Find other ways of getting companionship

➤ **Encourage the person you are caring for to call people on the telephone.**

The phone can be a means of keeping in touch with others when people are not able to visit. Encourage friends and loved ones to initiate phone calls, as well, but explain that the person you are caring for may not always feel up to talking on the phone.

➤ **Adopt a pet to provide companionship.**

Pets make wonderful friends and companions. People who are ill or who spend a great deal of time alone find pets to be a source of comfort and companionship. Pets have even been shown to have a therapeutic effect on some people. Ask your doctor if there are any possible health or safety problems for the person with HIV/AIDS that are associated with adopting a pet.

➤ **Encourage letter writing and card sending.**

Sending and receiving letters is another way of staying connected with people. Letter writing does not need to be demanding or mentally taxing: Most people would welcome short messages sent in cards that merely bring greetings and good wishes. Sending and receiving letters also gives the person you are caring for something to look forward to. If writing is not possible or enjoyable, messages can be recorded on audiotape and mailed.

4. POSSIBLE OBSTACLES TO CAREGIVING

Here are some common attitudes, fears, and misconceptions that may prevent you from carrying out your plan:

"People should want to visit without being asked."

Response: If you feel this way, think back to times when people you knew were sick and how difficult it sometimes was to find the time to visit. At other times, perhaps you did not call or visit because you were afraid of bothering them. The fact that people do not volunteer does not mean that they do not care. Probably they would welcome the opportunity to visit, if they were asked.

"I'm not sure who would be good company. What if I invite the wrong persons?"

Response: It is always safest to discuss visits and visitors with the person you are caring for. He or she knows who would be good company at a given time.

"Some people feel awkward talking to someone who is sick. They don't know what to say."

Response: Make sure that these people have something to do during the visit—a card game to play or a movie to watch. Then people can talk if they want to, or they can be involved in the activity. This puts the visitor and the person with HIV/AIDS more at ease.

"I don't want people to see me when I'm sick."

Response: Encourage him or her to talk to people on the phone. Also, consider inviting only those people who are comfortable being with sick people, such as people who have been caring for someone else with HIV/AIDS. You should also encourage conversations or activities that the visitors enjoy so that the person's appearance and illness are not the primary focus.

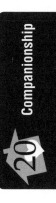

"Some people are 'well meaning,' but they try to tell me what to do and what not to do."

Response: So-called well-meaning people are not always helpful, so think carefully about when their visits would be welcome and when they would not. It is up to the both you and the person you are caring for to decide when people should visit and for how long. Before the well-meaning person comes over, you and the person with HIV/AIDS should make a plan in advance for steering any unwelcome conversations in a more positive direction.

"Some people stay too long and tire me out."

Response: Beforehand, ask people who usually stay too long to limit their stay. This takes the pressure off of everyone about when to end the visit.

Think of other obstacles

Identify additional roadblocks that could keep you from following the recommendations in this home care plan:

- Will the person I am caring for cooperate?
- Will other people help?
- How can I explain my needs to others?
- Do I have the time and energy to carry out this plan?

You need to develop plans for getting around these roadblocks. Use the four COPE ideas (Creativity, Optimism, Planning, and Expert information) in developing your plans. See pp 4–8 for a discussion of how to use the four COPE ideas in overcoming your obstacles.

5. CARRYING OUT AND ADJUSTING YOUR PLAN

Checking on results

You will know if your plans for companionship are successful by the number of times—either in person or on the phone—the person with HIV/AIDS is talking with other people. Make sure that he or she is happy doing this. If not, cut back on the number of visits.

What to do if your plan does not work

1. Review this chapter.

2. If you find that you've skipped something, try it now.

3. If you find that you've done all that you can, call the doctor for further guidance.

Try not to become discouraged if you are not successful at first. Keep discussing new ideas with the person you are caring for. You should repeat these problem-solving steps regularly throughout the illness to ensure that the person you are caring for has the companionship he or she wants and needs.

Community
Agencies

21

Getting Help from Community Agencies and Volunteer Groups

Overview of the Home Care Plan for
Getting Help from Community Agencies and Volunteer Groups

 1. UNDERSTANDING THE PROBLEM

> Learning about the availability of services in your community
>
> Your goals

 2. WHEN TO GET PROFESSIONAL HELP

> Symptoms that indicate the need for professional help
>
> What to say when you call

 3. WHAT YOU CAN DO TO GET HELP

> Getting help in finding community services
>
> Getting transportation
>
> Getting home nursing services
>
> Getting help with meals and household chores
>
> Getting hospice care
>
> Getting help with medical and hospital expenses
>
> Using community resources

 4. POSSIBLE OBSTACLES TO CAREGIVING

 5. CARRYING OUT AND ADJUSTING YOUR PLAN

> Carrying out your plan
>
> What to do if your plan does not work

Topics that have an arrow (➤) in front of them are actions you can take or symptoms you can look for.

Getting Help from Community Agencies and Volunteer Groups

1. UNDERSTANDING THE PROBLEM

Many people with HIV/AIDS and their caregivers may not know what services are available to help them in their own communities and in the hospitals where they receive treatment. As a result, they struggle alone with their problems when there are people and organizations able and willing to help. Finding out about these services and how to qualify for and use them is part of your job as a caregiver.

Even if you do not need to use these services right now, knowing that they are available is like "having money in the bank." It can reassure you that there are resources available to help when you need them.

Many types of services that persons with HIV/AIDS sometimes need and which are available in most communities are discussed in this chapter. They include transportation assistance, home care services, support groups, help with meals and household chores, and help paying medical or hospital expenses.

It is very helpful if you learn about available services *before* problems arise. You can do a more complete job of learning about available services before you are in the middle of a crisis. When you need the services, you will know what to do and where to go immediately.

> ➤ The information in this home care plan fits most situations, but yours may be different.
>
> ➤ If the doctor or nurse tells you to do something else, follow what he or she says.
>
> ➤ See the section "When To Get Professional Help" on p 246.

YOUR GOALS

Know when to get professional help to find services

Getting help in finding community services

Getting transportation

Getting home nursing services

Getting help with meals and household chores

Getting hospice care

Paying medical and hospital expenses

Using community resources

2. WHEN TO GET PROFESSIONAL HELP

If you or the person you are caring for feel helpless and that there is no help available, you should seek professional advice. Social workers are your primary source of help with these problems. It is their job to know what services are available in your community. Other professionals, such as nurses, doctors, and counselors, may also be able to help. (See "Getting Help in Finding Community Services" on pp 247–248 for a list of resources to call.) Call any one of these resources if any of the following situations is true:

➤ The person with HIV/AIDS feels like abandoning treatment because medical bills have become overwhelming.

➤ He or she is eating poorly because food shopping and meal preparation have become too hard to do.

➤ He or she needs special adaptive equipment in the home but does not know how to get it.

➤ You feel that you can no longer go on caring for person with HIV/AIDS in the home because health problems have become unmanageable.

➤ Getting to the clinic or hospital has become too difficult because of weakness or lack of transportation.

➤ You or the person you are caring for feels alone in his or her struggle with the disease.

➤ The person you are caring for has lost his or her job and health benefits.

Here is an example of what you might say when calling [a social worker] for professional help:

"This is Roberta Stone, Jane Smith's caregiver. Jane is a patient of Dr. Brown. She is very upset and wants to stop all of her clinic appointments and treatments. Jane worries about wearing me out as I try to care for her. She also doesn't think that others understand what she needs. She wants more help and support but doesn't know where and how to get it."

WHAT YOU CAN DO TO HELP

> ### THERE ARE MANY
> ### KINDS OF HELP AVAILABLE
>
> Help in finding community services
>
> Transportation assistance
>
> Home nursing services
>
> Help with meals and household chores
>
> Hospice care
>
> Help with paying medical and hospital expenses
>
> Community resources

Getting help in finding community services

Here are six places you can go for help in finding and using services in the community. Try all of these because one may list something that others do not.

> #### ➤ Hospital social workers or nurse discharge planners.

These are professionals with knowledge, skills, and experience in finding community services to help patients and their families deal with illness-related problems. They deal regularly with community agencies and know what services are available and which agencies provide the best services. You are entitled to talk to hospital social workers when the person you are caring for is a patient in the hospital or is coming for treatment at the hospital. Usually you can call the social workers directly without obtaining a referral, but some hospitals prefer that the doctor refer you. To get a referral, tell the doctor or nurse that you want to talk to a social worker.

> #### ➤ "Knowledgeable people" in your community.

Clergy or leaders of local HIV/AIDS community groups or support groups are usually well informed about which local agencies and organizations provide services. If these people cannot help you directly, they usually know who can.

➤ Agencies that help you find services.

Most communities have agencies that specialize in helping people find the services they need. The names of these agencies vary, depending on the part of the country that you are in. Every state has services available for persons with HIV/AIDS through their Department of Health Services. State or local health departments may be contacted. Community mental health centers, certain church-related groups, and community AIDS Service Organizations (ASOs) will also offer help.

➤ The "Guide to Human Services" section of local telephone books.

Most local telephone books list community agencies and the services they provide. Often these lists can be found in a separate section, often printed on a different-colored paper (usually blue) to set it off from the rest of the pages. Check the table of contents in the beginning of your local telephone book for the Guide to Human Services—or a similar title. You can also check the index to the yellow pages for the page numbers of the sections on Human Services Organizations and Social Service Organizations.

➤ The doctor's office or health care clinic.

Professionals in these settings know what services exist in the local community and can give you telephone numbers and information.

➤ AIDS Hotline.

Several hotlines have been set up across the country to answer questions about the disease, its treatment, and local resources.

HOTLINE NUMBERS*

National AIDS Hotline of the U.S. Centers for Disease Control and Prevention: **1-800-342-AIDS**

Project Inform: **1-800-822-7422**

National Institute of Drug Abuse Hotline: **1-800-662-HELP**

National Sexually Transmitted Disease Hotline: **1-800-227-8922**

National Child Abuse Hotline: **1-800-422-4453**

*See Appendix A (p 307) for more resources and telephone numbers.

Getting transportation

Getting transportation to and from treatments or medical appointments can be difficult. You should look for help if any of the following are true:

1. You cannot drive the person to appointments.

2. You cannot get the person from the house to the car, or he or she cannot sit for the length of the trip.

3. You are falling asleep at the wheel, the trip is too long, you hesitate to drive, or you fear the trip.

4. You cannot miss work or give up the wages to take the time needed for the trip, the waiting, the appointment, and the return trip.

Here are some steps you can take to solve these transportation problems:

➤ **Ask family or friends for help with driving.**

The more specific you are, the more likely it will be that others will understand your request and be able to judge whether they can help. Specific things to tell them include

What days of the week you need drivers

How long the trip takes each way

Whether the person you are caring for can be dropped off

Whether someone will meet the person you are caring for at the door

The cost of parking

How long the usual appointment lasts

Whether he or she needs help getting in and out of the car

Whether a wheelchair is involved

➤ **Ask someone else to arrange help with transportation.**

If you do not want to ask for help, have someone else ask for you. Having a scheduler is especially helpful when the person you are caring for must go for treatments or clinic appointments on a regular basis.

➤ **Inquire about volunteer transportation services in your area.**

Call your local community AIDS Service Organization (ASO) to ask about transportation. Volunteers who are trained to help persons who are ill during transportation may be available for you. Their services are usually free.

➤ **Call local agencies to inquire about eligibility requirements for reimbursement for gas or cab fares.**

Local AIDS programs, the American Cancer Society, the Hemophilia Society, and the Leukemia Society (helping those persons with AIDS who have lymphoma) can be called to explore the availability of funds for transportation to and from hospitals and clinics.

Getting home nursing services

Three types of nursing services can be considered:

➤ **Visits from registered nurses.**

A doctor can prescribe home visits by registered nurses to do skilled nursing procedures and to give certain treatments within the home. Registered nurses can do procedures in the home such as taking blood and urine samples, giving daily treatments or IV medications, helping with dressing changes on a wound, or caring for an IV site. Nurses can come several times during the week to do "skilled nursing procedures," such as teaching the person with HIV/AIDS or the caregiver how to care for an IV catheter, change a dressing on a wound, or take medicines correctly. Their visits are often short (about an hour), and the cost is generally covered by insurance, if preapproved by the doctor and insurance company. Visiting nurses can often arrange for other services, if needed, such as visits from nurse's aides, social workers, speech therapists, occupational therapists, and physical therapists.

➤ **Visits from private duty nurses.**

You can arrange for private duty nurses without a doctor's approval by calling a professional nursing service organization. Visits from private duty nurses can last as long as you want. Some families find it helpful to arrange for 8 hours of overnight care by a private duty nurse. The cost of this service can be expensive and is usually not covered by health insurance. Private duty nurses can be registered nurses, licensed practical nurses, or nurse's aides. Their services are available through professional nursing service organizations within the local community.

➤ **Visits from home health aides, sitters, companions.**

You can arrange for nurse's aides, sitters, or companions to provide personal care services within the home. The services of a home health aide or nurse's aide will be supervised by a registered nurse from the same agency. If you arrange for sitters or companions on your own, you will have to supervise them.

Sitters or companions have some degree of experience caring for those who are ill. They stay with the sick person for varying amounts of time (2 to 24 hours) during a given day, offering assistance and companionship.

Getting help with meals and household chores

➤ **Homemaker services.**

These services provide someone to shop, clean, run errands, and prepare meals for the person who is ill. Sometimes these services are available free from volunteer groups, and sometimes they must be paid for. Ask for help from a social worker, nurse, or other professional when selecting the service or agency, because some are better than others.

➤ **Home-delivered meals.**

Ask your social worker or nurse discharge planner about programs offering home-delivered meals. Most cities and towns have Meals-on-Wheels programs, which deliver meals to the home of the person who is housebound. Many of these programs are for senior citizens, but others may still be able to qualify. Call and ask. The cost of the service varies, and some people are eligible for reduced rates. Usually, a hot lunch is delivered with a cold meal to be eaten later in the day. Special diets are available, such as diabetic, kosher, low-sodium, and low-fat diets.

➤ **Ask church groups or neighbors to function as a home helper group.**

Accept help from church members or neighbors. Many churches are happy to do this. Members often will do yard work, window washing, or other chores. Sometimes they arrange that the youth group get involved. Neighbors are often willing to help with grocery shopping, picking up prescriptions, and occasionally providing transportation.

Getting hospice care

Ask the social worker or nurse about hospice care in your community. Hospice teams help people with life-limiting or terminal illnesses near the end of life. Their services are available in all cities and most towns and rural areas. Hospices are often run by the local visiting nurse agencies, and hospice team visits are covered by insurance. Nurses and social workers at the hospital or clinics where the person receives treatment will know whom to call about hospice care, and a hospice worker can talk with you about their many services.

Getting help with medical and hospital expenses

It is important that you deal with financial problems early, before a crisis arises. Do not put off doing so. The earlier you start working on financial problems, the easier they will be to solve. If you talk to the people to whom you owe money before it becomes a serious credit problem, they are usually willing to work with you. The following is a list of suggestions for solving problems paying medical or hospital bills.

➤ Collect information about medical expenses.

First, collect information about the medical expenses. Make a list of all of the financial resources of the person you are caring for. This information will be needed to determine what help is needed and to determine the person's eligibility for financial assistance. Having information about bills, monthly expenses, and available funds will help expedite the process. Find out:

1. How much does the person you are caring for currently owe for medical expenses? This is often difficult to determine on your own, especially with the confusing way that many hospitals and other health care organizations bill for services. Most hospitals and doctors' offices have staff members who understand the billing forms. These people can quickly go through a stack of bills and determine exactly what a person owes at that time.

2. What future expenses are anticipated? Knowing present expenses can sometimes help in predicting future expenses.

3. Approximately how much has been paid out so far for medical care during this illness? Keep an accurate account of medical expenses that are not covered by insurance because they may be tax-deductible. This information will help show others that financial assistance is needed.

➤ Determine the person's financial resources.

1. Which medical expenses are paid for by insurance and which are not? This is very important information to have even before the bills arrive because it helps in estimating what expenses the person will have to pay himself or herself. Ask the insurance agent or health insurance representative what the policy covers.

2. Does the person you are caring for have any savings plans?

3. What assets does the person have (house, property, stocks)?

4. What is the total income for the household? Household income is the total income of everyone living in the same household with the person who is ill. This information is

often used to determine whether the person with HIV/AIDS is eligible for financial assistance.

➤ **Investigate spacing out payments or paying bills in installments.**

To find out about spacing out payments, contact the financial counselor or the business or credit office in the hospital. A monthly payment plan can be arranged. Some hospitals, doctors, and pharmacies will submit bills to the insurance company and then bill for what the insurance will not pay. This saves one from paying the bills and then waiting for reimbursement from the insurance company. Ask the hospital or doctor's office if they will do this.

➤ **Apply for financial aid.**

If the person with HIV/AIDS no longer has a job, it is possible that he or she no longer has health insurance. If this is the case, financial assistance and insurance coverage of some sort is a must. Social workers are usually the best source of information on how to get help with medical expenses and on who qualifies for assistance. All health care agencies have social workers as well as financial counselors on their staffs.

In the United States, Medicaid, which is administered by each state's department of public assistance, will pay the medical bills of qualified persons. Qualifications include low income and limited financial resources. The exact requirements change periodically and vary from one state to another. Therefore, you should contact your local department of public assistance, which is listed in your telephone directory, to learn whether the person you are caring for qualifies for Medicaid assistance. You can also ask your social worker for the address and telephone number.

Help with medication costs is sometimes available through grants and funds provided by the pharmaceutical companies that produce the drugs used to treat AIDS. The Burroughs Wellcome Co., for example, produces the drug AZT (also known as Zidovudine), widely used in the treatment of HIV/AIDS. Persons with HIV/AIDS who enter clinical drug trials will usually have some of their medication expenses covered. Some states offer help obtaining medicine used to treat HIV/AIDS. Call your local or state department of health for more information and ask your physician or social worker about how to get financial assistance for medication.

If you live in Canada, talk to your social worker about sources of help or call the Canada AIDS Society for information (1-613-230-3580) for information and guidance in obtaining financial help for persons with HIV/AIDS.

Using community resources

Many national and state agencies are available to inform persons with HIV/AIDS about available resources.

STATE AND NATIONAL AGENCIES*

➤ The American Foundation for AIDS Research (AMFAR). Telephone: (212) 333-3118 or (213) 273-5547. This agency supports clinical research projects, provides community education, and publishes a treatment directory.

➤ National AIDS Hotline of the U.S. Centers for Disease Control and Prevention: 1-800-342-AIDS.

➤ The Centers for Disease Control and Prevention— AIDS Activity Project. Telephone: (404) 639-2891. This agency offers educational materials, a listing of HIV testing sites, and national reports on the disease of AIDS.

➤ The Fund for Human Dignity. Telephone: (212) 529-1600 or 1-800-221-7044 (crisis line). This agency offers counseling and referral information (A National Directory of AIDS-Related Services and AIDS Service Agencies).

➤ Gay Men's Health Crisis. Telephone: (212) 807-6655. This agency offers legal aid, financial aid, housing, counseling, and educational information.

***See Appendix A (p 307) for more resources and telephone numbers.**

Most communities have many AIDS projects and task forces. Please refer to the human service directory in your telephone book under HIV/AIDS, or call a hospital social worker or nurse discharge planner to find these services. Another source of information about local support services is your local or state department of health. There are also international programs that have been developed by and that are encouraged by the World Health Organization (WHO), located in Geneva, Switzerland. Call 011-412-291-2673 to learn about these international programs.

See Appendices A and B (pp 307–310) for listings of local, state, and national resources in the United States and Canada.

LOCAL SUPPORT SERVICES*

➤ DC AIDS Task Force. Telephone: (202) 332-5295 or (202) 332-EXAM (HIV testing line). This service offers counseling, support groups, an IV drug program, legal aid, transportation, and more.

➤ AIDS Institute of New York. Telephone: (212) 340-3388. This service offers housing, community education, legal aid, counseling, and HIV testing sites information.

➤ Seattle AIDS Action Project. Telephone: (206) 323-1229. This service offers AIDS testing, counseling, support groups, and direct service referrals.

➤ PWA (People With AIDS) Coalition in New York City. Telephone: (212) 566-4995. This service offers community education, support groups for AIDS patients and women with AIDS, experimental treatment information, and the handbook "Striving and Thriving with AIDS."

➤ AIDS Services of Chicago. Telephone: (312) 871-5777. This service offers counseling; support groups for patients, others, and the worried well; buddies; testing for HIV; legal referrals; and speakers on the topic of AIDS.

➤ Baltimore Health Education Resource Organization (HERO). Telephone: (410) 945-AIDS. This service offers community and professional education, support groups, buddies, housing, transportation, prison outreach, minority outreach, and financial help.

➤ Philadelphia AIDS Task Force. Telephone: (215) 545-8686. This service offers housing for PWAs, HIV testing and counseling, education, and medical and dental referrals.

➤ AIDS Foundation of Houston. Telephone: (713) 623-6796. This service offers a buddy program, counseling on legal affairs, support groups for PWAs and health care workers, food and clothing bank, physician referral, financial assistance, rent assistance, and transportation.

*The list is not complete but these groups can also connect you to a support service near where you live. See also Appendix A (p 307) for more resources and telephone numbers.

Community Agencies

21

4. POSSIBLE OBSTACLES TO CAREGIVING

Here are some common attitudes, fears, and misconceptions that may prevent you from carrying out your plan:

"I don't know anyone around here who can help drive. They don't have the time or the money for gas. Some don't even have cars. They work or are too busy with their families."

Response: You don't know who can drive until you ask. Ask other people to help you find drivers. Also, retirees and those who are temporarily unemployed might have the time to give to help you solve this problem.

"I'd rather not go for my treatments, even though I need them. I don't want to use up my insurance benefits."

Response: *Now* is the time to use those benefits—during a serious illness. Some policies do have maximum benefits, but the maximum is usually quite high. Check the insurance policy to be sure, or apply for financial assistance if this becomes necessary. If the insurance coverage is exhausted, the person you are caring for may qualify for Medicaid. Call your local office of public assistance to learn if he or she qualifies.

"I feel embarrassed not to be able to pay my bills."

Response: Many other people have been in the same situation. Medical expenses are so high today that it is becom-

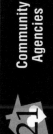
ing common for people to have problems paying them. Assure the person that there is no reason for embarrassment.

"I didn't handle money in our family. Other people always did this for me, so I don't know what to do."

Response: If money matters are new to you, then get help from someone who is familiar with budgets and paying bills. Don't let things drift, because then they can get out of hand and you will have a financial crisis to deal with.

Think of other obstacles

Identify additional roadblocks that could keep you from following the recommendations in this home care plan:

- Will the person I am caring for cooperate?

- Will other people help?

- How can I explain my needs to others?

- Do I have the time and energy to carry out this plan?

You need to develop plans for getting around these roadblocks. Use the four COPE ideas (Creativity, Optimism, Planning and Expert information) in developing your plans. See pp 4–8 for a discussion of how to use the four COPE ideas in overcoming your obstacles.

5. CARRYING OUT AND ADJUSTING YOUR PLAN

Carrying out your plan

Don't wait! Start learning now about how community agencies and service groups can help you. This will be valuable information that you can use when you need it. If you have trouble getting the information you need, ask someone to help you. Talk to a social worker or a nurse discharge planner at the hospital. They have had a great deal of experience with these problems and can often be creative in helping you to get the help you need.

What to do if your plan does not work

1. Review this chapter.

2. If you find that you've skipped something, try it now.

If you are having some success but not as much as you would like, you may be expecting too much progress too soon. Be patient and keep trying. It often takes time to learn how to use community agencies and service groups.

If you are feeling worn down by your problems, ask someone else to help you work out a solution. Sometimes people who are not directly involved can see new ways to deal with a problem.

Social workers are the professionals who have the most experience with these problems. If the social worker to whom you talked was not helpful, ask to talk to another social worker.

Getting Treatment Information
(Including Alternative Treatments)

22

Overview of the Home Care Plan for
Getting Treatment Information
(Including Alternative Treatments)

 1. *UNDERSTANDING THE PROBLEM*

Difficulties in getting medical information

Learning the kinds of information that different health professionals can give you

Your goals

2. *GETTING INFORMATION IN AN EMERGENCY*

Whom to call for help

What to say when you call

3. *IMPROVING YOUR ABILITY TO GET INFORMATION*

Be sure that your questions are phrased clearly

Learn who can answer your questions

Ask your questions yourself or have someone else ask the questions for you

Getting information on alternative treatments

Ask questions about alternative treatments

4. *POSSIBLE OBSTACLES TO CAREGIVING*

 5. *CARRYING OUT AND ADJUSTING YOUR PLAN*

Carrying out your plan

Checking on results

What to do if your plan does not work

> **Topics that have an arrow (➤) in front of them are actions you can take or symptoms you can look for.**

Getting Treatment Information (Including Alternative Treatments)

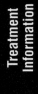

1. UNDERSTANDING THE PROBLEM

Over the course of this illness, you will need a great deal of information to help you in your caregiver role. Some of this information is complicated, and often it must come from different sources. It is not surprising that many caregivers experience problems getting the information that they need at some time during the illness. This chapter will help you to deal with this problem by giving you suggestions on how to get the medical information that you and the person you are caring for need.

There are two things you should bear in mind about getting medical information:

1. *It is reasonable to assume that health professionals (doctors, nurses, and social workers) want to help you and would like to give you the information you need.*

2. *It may be necessary to talk with many health care professionals to get the information you need.* Each professional person has his or her special area of knowledge. This can make getting information difficult. It can even seem confusing at times. Part of your job as a caregiver is to learn who can give you the kinds of information that you need.

Sometimes the information will be too technical to understand. If so, ask for someone to explain the information to you in terms you understand.

> ➤ The information in this home care plan fits most situations, but yours may be different.
>
> ➤ If the doctor or nurse tells you to do something else, follow what he or she says.

If you or the patient do not speak English well, it would be helpful to bring someone with you to interpret information. You may also ask the nurse or social worker if an interpreter is available.

Kinds of information that different health professionals can give you

Physicians can give you information on treatment plans, how often the patient needs to see the doctor, when a hospital admission is necessary, what medications should be taken and when, test results, and the effects of treatments on the disease.

Nurses can give information on medications, the management of side effects of treatments or medications, nutrition information, ways of maintaining comfort and quality of life, and clarification of physician's orders.

Social workers or nurse discharge planners can give information on how to obtain help in dealing with social and emotional problems; how to arrange for medical care or equipment at home, in a nursing home, or in a hospice; financial assistance and counseling; and support for coping with the illness.

Physicians with different titles and specialties will have different responsibilities and will be able to tell you different kinds of information. If several physicians are involved, one will be coordinating the care. In this case, you should ask who the coordinating physician is.

YOUR GOALS

Know how to get information in an emergency

Be sure that your questions are phrased clearly

Learn who can answer your questions

Ask yourself or have someone ask for you

Get information on alternative treatments

Ask questions about alternative treatments

---

2. GETTING INFORMATION IN AN EMERGENCY

Whom to call for help

If you feel that the person you are caring for is having a medical emergency, you should call the doctor, the clinic, or an emergency room. Be sure the person to whom you speak understands that you feel this is an emergency. *Use the word "emergency" in your question and then be persistent until you have the information you need.*

Here are examples of what you might say when calling for professional help in the event of an emergency

"I have an emergency and need to talk to a doctor."

(Be prepared to answer the question "What is the emergency?")

"I have a question about _____ , and I'm not sure if it this is really an emergency or not. Who can help me?"

"I'm very concerned about _____ . I think it may be an emergency. Can you help me?"

Have a special place where you keep important phone numbers and the names of people you may need to contact in an emergency. Having a phone list that is kept near the telephone is very helpful. Also keep a copy of the list in your purse or wallet.

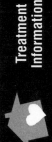

 ## IMPROVING YOUR ABILITY TO GET INFORMATION

> ### HERE ARE FIVE STEPS YOU CAN TAKE TO IMPROVE YOUR ABILITY TO GET INFORMATION:
>
> Follow these steps in the order listed below:
>
> 1. Be sure that your questions are phrased clearly.
>
> 2. Learn who can answer your questions.
>
> 3. Ask your questions yourself or have someone else ask the questions for you
>
> 4. Get information on alternative treatments
>
> 6. Ask questions about alternative treatments

Be sure that your questions are phrased clearly

Know exactly what information you need and state your questions clearly.

➤ **Ask yourself "What do I need to know to help the person who is ill?"**

This question focuses your attention on what is important and on the questions that should be asked. For example, you might decide that you want to know: What is the stage of the illness? How often do people continue to work or feel well with the disease at this stage? Are options available for other medical treatments? Think about what you *and* the person with HIV/AIDS need to know to cope with the illness.

➤ **When you ask a question, state *what* you need to know and then *why* you need to know it.**

It is much easier for someone else to understand your question if you start with a clear statement of the information you need. Here is an example:

"This is Peter Smith, John Mitchell's caregiver. John Mitchell is a patient of Dr. Black. John has been running a fever of 101 °F every afternoon that is usually gone by the next morning. Should we be concerned about this? We are worried because he just recovered from a kidney infection, and we are concerned that it is coming back."

➤ **Write out your questions so you will not forget to ask them.**

Writing down your questions ahead of time is a sure way to get all of them asked and to ask them clearly.

Learn who can answer your questions

Different people will be able to give you different kinds of information. *You need to know who can tell you the different kinds of information you need for each new treatment setting.*

➤ **Learn which staff members give which kinds of information.**

The best way to learn which staff members give which kinds of information is to ask a medical staff person such as a nurse, social worker, or physician. Secretarial staff are less likely to know how to get this information, but sometimes they can be helpful. Start by asking a nurse or social worker, "Who can tell me . . . " For example, "Who can tell me when my husband will be discharged?" or "Who can tell me when my mother's treatments are scheduled?"

Be prepared to learn the rules about who can give you what information for every new group of health staff that you deal with. It is a good idea to ask these questions early—as soon as you begin working with a new treatment team.

➤ **Be persistent!**

If the persons you ask do not have the information you need, then ask them if they know who does. Secretaries, clerks, and schedulers often do not have the detailed information you need or want. You may have to ask several people before your questions are answered. Remember the medical care system can be complicated, so do not become discouraged. You have a right to get all of the information that you need.

Persistence almost always pays off. Getting information becomes easier and easier the better you understand the medical care system.

Ask your questions yourself or have someone else ask the questions for you

The person you are caring for may not want to ask his or her own questions about treatment, the illness, or existing symptoms. Often this is because of fear that the information will be upsetting. In this case, you should take the lead and get the information that you both need.

> ➤ **Ask your questions yourself.**

Have a clear idea what you need to know, ask or read your questions, and ask follow-up questions until you are very clear about the answer you received.

> ➤ **Ask a nurse, social worker, or other member of the health care team to get the information you need.**

You may need to ask someone else to get information for you because you do not have the time to find the right person. This could be because the medical person you need to talk to is not available when you need the information, or it could be that he or she gives you an answer that is unclear or does not give you the information you need. In these cases, a good strategy is to ask a nurse or social worker to ask your questions for you. Choose nurses or social workers with whom you feel comfortable, and tell them what information you need and why you cannot get it yourself. Then ask for their help.

Ask questions about alternative treatments

In addition to conventional medical treatments, there are "alternative" ways of treating HIV/AIDS and of feeling better. Some of the many different alternative treatments include diets, herbs, and unofficial HIV medicines, as well as body therapies, such as coffee enemas, relaxation, biofeedback, and acupuncture.

Claims are made of these treatments—some are true, many are not. Some claim to decrease side effects, improve the quality of life, or improve chances of surviving the disease. These treatments represent a very mixed bag of choices. They differ in their effectiveness, in their acceptance by the medical community, in their cost, and in their availability.

Although some of these treatments may be helpful, you should remind the person with HIV/AIDS to be careful and not let the stress of dealing with the disease affect his or her judgment as a wise consumer. *If someone claims miraculous results, be skeptical.*

Your doctors may or may not be familiar with some alternative treatments but, as professionals, they should be open to discussing them. The person you are caring for should also be honest about what alternative treatments he or she is using or planning to use. Some alternative treatments can *interfere* with the "mainstream" therapies for HIV/AIDS. Mainstream therapies are those treatments that have been experimentally tested and that are given by doctors.

Some practitioners of alternative medicine strongly oppose all forms of conventional medical care and urge persons with HIV/AIDS to discontinue all conventional medical therapy. If the person you are caring for is considering discontinuing prescribed medicines, it is best to discuss this with the doctor. Maybe the person with HIV/AIDS can take both types of treatments—the medical ones and the alternative ones.

Questions you should ask when considering alternative treatments are

- Will the alternative treatment interfere with the regular treatments? (If so, urge the person you are caring for to talk openly with the doctor about it.)

- Is the alternate treatment safe, or could it actually cause harm?

- If the alterative treatment is used, will he or she be glad to have tried it, even if it does not produce the promised effect? (For example, will it make the person more relaxed, or help him or her to feel more "in control" of the treatment plan?)

Some examples of safe treatments include

- Meditation, relaxation, or prayer. Often people who have left an organized religion still find that prayer gives them a feeling of peace.

- Improving one's diet in a conventional way—for example, reducing fat and cholesterol intake

- Exercise

- Seeking support and friends through support groups or new relationships

Choose only those alternative treatments that do not interfere with regular medical treatments and are comfortable and not forced. If the person you are caring for needs to force himself or herself to take part in an alternative treatment or if it feels uncomfortable, then it is probably not something that he or she will be happy with.

 4. POSSIBLE OBSTACLES TO CAREGIVING

Here are some common attitudes, fears, and misconceptions that may prevent you from carrying out your plan:

"I'm afraid to ask questions because I think that my questions may sound stupid."

Response: No question is stupid. You and the health care professionals want to give the best possible care to the person with HIV/AIDS. To accomplish this, you must understand what you need to do and why. Therefore *it is the job of health care professionals* to educate and inform you.

"I feel confused by the health care system."

Response: Health care professionals may use unfamiliar words, leaving persons with HIV/AIDS and their caregivers overwhelmed by the "new language." This can be almost as confusing as going to a foreign country. What many people do when they go to a foreign country is get a guide who speaks both their language and the language of the new country. This is a good model for learning about the health care system. *Your guides can be health care staff who know the system. Nurses and social workers are often good guides.* Ask them to explain the system to you.

"I feel intimidated by health care professionals."

Response: Some people feel that health care professionals are busy and that they should not take up their valuable time with questions. *Remember: Health professionals are there to help patients.* To do this, they need to give caregivers the information they need. Good health professionals do not look down on you and the person you care for because he or she has HIV/AIDS. Their job is to help you to get the information and assistance you need.

"If I need to know something, the doctor will tell me."

Response: This is not necessarily true! Although your doctor will try to tell you everything you need to know, he or she cannot always remember what you were told before, may assume that someone else has already told you, or may simply forget to tell you certain things.

"If I ask too many questions, the staff will think I am a nuisance, and then they won't take good care of the person I am caring for. "

Response: It is unlikely that staff will think that you are a nuisance but, even if they do, there is no reason to fear that this would affect how they treat the person you are caring for. Health care professionals are trained to treat everyone to the best of their ability, giving them whatever care is needed.

Think of other obstacles

Identify additional roadblocks that could keep you from following the recommendations in this home care plan:

- Will the person I am caring for cooperate?
- Will other people help?
- How can I explain my needs to others?
- Do I have te time and energy to carry out this plan?

You need to develop plans for getting around these roadblocks. Use the four COPE ideas (*Creativity, Optimism, Planning,* and *Expert information*) in developing your plans. See pp 4–8 for a discussion of how to use the four COPE ideas in overcoming your obstacles.

5. CARRYING OUT AND ADJUSTING YOUR PLANS

Carrying out your plan

Be persistent in asking questions. *The more questions you ask, the easier it becomes.* In the beginning, you may want to read your questions. Also, practice beforehand what you will say. Set deadlines for when you will get certain information.

Checking on results

Keep track of the number of times you have problems getting information you need, as well as the number of times that you succeed. Do not expect perfect results right away. However, over time, you should notice significant improvement in your ability to get information you need.

What to do if your plan does not work

1. Review this chapter.

2. If you find that you've skipped something, try it now.

3. If you are having some success but not as much as you would like, you may be expecting too much progress too soon. Be patient and keep trying. The medical care system is complicated, so it will take time to master it.

4. If you feel that medical staff are not giving you the information you need, your next step should be to make an appointment with the coordinating physician (the one who has primary responsibility for the patient's care at that time). Ask him or her your questions. You should also explain the problems you have had in getting information and ask how to avoid these problems in the future.

   (Note that you may be charged for this appointment and that many insurers will not pay for appointments between physicians and caregivers. It is best to ask about this when making the appointment. If you cannot afford to pay, you can ask to have the fee waived or you can ask if your meeting can be scheduled as part of the patient's regular meeting with the physician.)

5. Most hospitals have patient advocates or persons in similar positions. These people are familiar with problems in their hospitals as well as with how to deal with those problems. They can give you guidance and help in getting information. They can also help to change the way the hospital operates. By contacting patient advocates with your problems, you may actually be able to help future patients avoid the problems you are having.

6. The person with HIV/AIDS has the right to change doctors or treatment settings if he or she is uncomfortable with the current doctor or treatment setting. If he or she is thinking of changing, be sure that the new setting will give the support that he or she wants and needs.

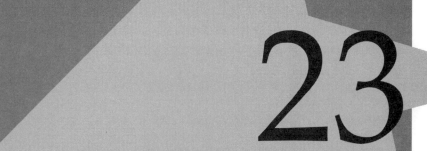

23

Substance Abuse

Overview of the Home Care Plan for *Substance Abuse*

 1. UNDERSTANDING THE PROBLEM

The problem of substance abuse

Substance abuse among persons with HIV/AIDS

Characteristics of persons with substance abuse problems

Effects of substance abuse on the person with HIV/AIDS

Your goals

 2. WHEN TO GET PROFESSIONAL HELP

Symptoms of substance abuse

 3. WHAT YOU CAN DO TO HELP

Avoid nagging and preaching

Encourage honesty and positive thinking

Promote self-affirmation

Support the process of change

 4. POSSIBLE OBSTACLES

5. CARRYING OUT AND ADJUSTING YOUR PLAN

Carrying out your plan

Checking on results

What to do if your plan does not work

Encourage the person to seek professional help

> **Topics that have an arrow (➤) in front of them are actions you can take or symptoms you can look for.**

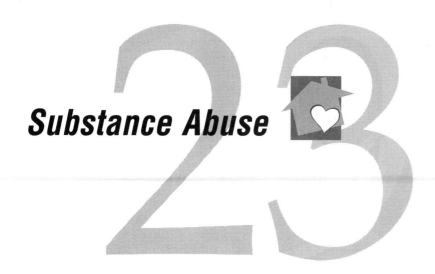

Substance Abuse

1. UNDERSTANDING THE PROBLEM

Unfortunately, substance abuse is a common problem in our society. Substance abusers depend on chemicals to help them cope with the problems, stresses, and responsibilities of life. They feel that, with the help of chemicals, whether drugs or alcohol, they will be better able to cope. This is far from true. The more entrapped individuals become in their substance abuse, the less responsible they are for their life choices, decisions, relationships, commitments, and problems.

Many persons with HIV/AIDS have had problems with substance abuse or chemical dependency. IV drug users account for the second largest group of HIV-positive persons. People with HIV/AIDS who are substance abusers may use drugs or alcohol to deal with the diagnosis and the fears regarding progression of the disease. However, the substance abuser learns all too soon that once the effects of the chemicals are gone, so are the false feelings of control. In their place

> ➤ The information in this home care plan fits most situations, but yours may be different.
>
> ➤ If the doctor or nurse tells you to do something else, follow what he or she says.
>
> ➤ See the section "When To Get Professional Help" on pp 275–278.

are left the fears, the feelings of helplessness, and the uncertainties about one's life, well-being, and future that come with the disease.

Substance abuse is a chronic, progressive disease that is characterized by the following factors:

- An inability to control one's use of a chemical substance

- The need to have that chemical substance to cope

- The need for greater and greater quantities of the chemical substance to feel "in control" or "on top of things"

- The continued use of the chemical substance despite the negative effects it is having on one's life, personality, health, family and relationships, job, and actions as a human being

Substance abuse usually begins as a social habit. This is easy in our society, in which smoking and alcohol use are socially acceptable practices. Using drugs or alcohol socially progresses to using them to cope at times of stress. Finally, dependence on them becomes an everyday problem. Periods of excessive use or bingeing may be followed by maintenance use. People with substance abuse problems soon feel the cost of their expensive habit. They may get in trouble with the law. Family members may leave them. Costs become increasingly higher when multiple drugs are in use (polydrug use).

Chemically dependent people begin to realize the high financial costs when they are forced to empty savings accounts, sell valuables, steal, or prostitute themselves. What they do not realize is that many other losses follow, including loss of a job, of family and trusted friends, of home and car, of health, and a total loss of control over one's life.

If the substance abuser has HIV/AIDS, problems increase steadily. The chemicals, whether drugs or alcohol, have a harmful effect not only on the body but also on the immune system, which is already being damaged by the AIDS virus. Substance abuse makes the person more vulnerable to a progression of the disease. It also makes the person more susceptible to infections caused by organisms other than the AIDS virus.

Sometimes the caregiver has lived a long time with the substance abuse problem. The person with HIV/AIDS may have kept his or her substance abuse problem reasonably well under control before the diagnosis, or the caregiver may have learned ways to cope with the problem. After the diagnosis, however, past coping behaviors need to be reviewed and the caregiver may need to learn how to help the person with HIV/AIDS limit or stop all substance abuse. Often, help or guidance from health professionals is needed to make this change.

> ## YOUR GOALS
>
> Get professional help when it is needed
>
> Avoid nagging and preaching
>
> Encourage honesty and positive thinking
>
> Promote self-affirmation
>
> Support the process of change

2. WHEN TO GET PROFESSIONAL HELP

If substance abuse is suspected in the person with HIV/AIDS, professional help may be needed. Substance abuse, if not treated, can cause the disease of AIDS to progress more rapidly by lowering the person's resistance and making him or her more vulnerable to increased infections.

Call the doctor or nurse if you notice behaviors that lead you to think that the person you are caring for is abusing drugs or alcohol

> ➤ It has become very hard to relate to the person you are caring for because of increased irritability, mood swings, and unsuspected outbursts of anger or laughter.
>
> ➤ He or she is often argumentative, accusing, or suspicious.
>
> ➤ You have a clear sense that he or she is lying to you most of the time, acts like he or she is hiding something, and gets angry when you ask questions about his or her behavior.
>
> ➤ His or her energy level changes drastically from sluggish and slow to hyperactive and agitated during the same day.
>
> ➤ The person you are caring for cares less about his or her appearance, about meeting responsibilities, and about keeping promises and commitments.
>
> ➤ He or she is spending time with different types of friends.
>
> ➤ You have noticed a significant change in his or her thinking ability—thoughts are either racing and scattered, or he or she is trying to cover up memory lapses and confused thinking.
>
> ➤ The person you are caring for is secretive about where he or she goes, how he or she is spending time during the day or night, with whom he or she is meeting, and how he or she is spending money.

Substance Abuse

23

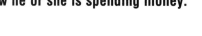

➤ **The person you are caring for is physically abusing you or others.**

If the person with HIV/AIDS is using a particular chemical substance, you will notice characteristic signs that should lead you to consult a professional for help. However, do not assume that the person you are caring for is a substance abuser simply because he or she exhibits the characteristic signs listed above. He or she may be suffering from depression or from AIDS dementia complex. (For a more detailed discussion of the signs and symptoms of these problems, see the home care plans "Coping with Depression" [Chapter 17] and "AIDS Dementia Complex" [Chapter 15].)

In addition to the above-mentioned signs of substance abuse, there are signs you can look for that are specific to alcohol abuse, depressant abuse, stimulant abuse, narcotics abuse, and hallucinogen abuse.

Signs of alcohol abuse

1. Frequent drinks are needed to get through the stresses of the day.

2. The person is defensive about drinking and denies drinking too much even when it is obvious that he or she is intoxicated.

3. The person drinks alone or sneaks drinks in order to hide how much alcohol he or she is using.

4. Behavior is restless and irritable. You may notice unsteadiness and shakiness, especially in the hands.

5. The person is irresponsible in caring for his or her appearance, nutrition, and commitments to others.

6. "Blackouts" or periods of not remembering what happened while intoxicated become more frequent.

Denial is a common defense used by the person who is abusing alcohol. He or she thinks that lying will cover up the drinking problem. He or she will deny being drunk, and the person may manipulate the caregiver into believing that he or she is exaggerating the whole situation. Alcoholic stupors and blackouts may occur, which are frightening to witness. Even in the midst of these, the person with the alcohol abuse problem will deny and lie. Nothing seems to be able to stop the excessive alcohol use.

Signs of depressant abuse

1. Behavior greatly resembles that of the alcohol abuser, but without the odor of alcohol on the breath.

2. The person staggers or stumbles.

3. Falling asleep or "nodding off" during the day becomes more common.

4. Speech becomes slurred, and he or she has difficulty concentrating.

Depressants commonly abused include sedatives, tranquilizers, and sleep medications. These medications are used to calm the nerves, ease "shakes," control fears and anxieties, and to "come down" after a high feeling caused by stimulants such as cocaine. When a person starts mixing drugs or classes of drugs, the problems become more serious. Using a combination of drugs has a more destructive effect on the immune system, as well as disturbs the chemical balance within the brain itself.

Signs of stimulant abuse

1. The person becomes nervous and "edgy."

2. The person is excessively active and has a great deal of energy. He or she talks more than usual, gets excited easily, and may even claim to be feeling "high" or "great."

3. The person may go for long periods without eating or sleeping.

4. The pupils are dilated (larger), the heartbeat is faster, and the blood pressure is usually high.

5. After a period of excitement and energy, the person experiences a "crash" of energy, and he or she may become depressed, distraught, or agitated.

Stimulants greatly energize the person who uses them by speeding up the body's whole inner workings (metabolism). During the "high" caused by the drugs, worries and problems seem to disappear. The person feels on top of things. However, after the effects of the drug wear off, mood and energy level rapidly become low (often lower than they were before the drug was used). This creates an urgent need for more of the drug. Cocaine and amphetamines (speed) are the most commonly used stimulants.

Signs of narcotics abuse

1. The person has scars from injecting narcotics such as heroin.

2. He or she feels no physical or emotional pain for a limited time, becomes drowsy, and often falls asleep.

3. The person is restless, sniffles, yawns, and has red, watery eyes when the level of the drug in the body drops. These symptoms disappear when the next dose of the narcotic is taken.

4. The pupils are constricted (small).

5. If the person is injecting narcotics, you may find needles, syringes, or other types of drug paraphernalia.

Commonly used narcotics include opium, methadone, heroin, and pain medications such as morphine, meperidine (Demerol), codeine, Percocet, and Percodan. These substances may be taken in tablet form or may be injected. Because the tablets take longer to act, the injectable forms of the drugs are often preferred. Heroin is one of the most commonly used narcotics because of its easy availability.

Signs of hallucinogen abuse

1. Mood and behavior vary widely with hallucinogens, but they are always extreme: The person may sit or lie in a trancelike state, become elated, fearful, or even terrified.

2. The person may make comments indicating that he or she is experiencing altered perceptions—for example, changes in hearing, sight, touch, smell, or sense of time.

3. The person may have difficulty communicating, organizing thoughts, and controlling his or her emotions.

4. The person may experience nausea, chills, irregular breathing, trembling, or sweating while under the influence of the drug.

Commonly used hallucinogens include LSD, PCP, and mescaline. These substances have a dramatic effect on the person using them. Feelings and moods are very often distorted. The experience can be pleasant and exciting, or it can be terrifying. The person may describe an "out of body" experience or being immersed in a sea of sound and color. The most devastating result of hallucinogen abuse is the long-term damaging effects these chemicals have on the brain and how the mind functions.

3. WHAT YOU CAN DO TO HELP

HERE ARE FOUR STEPS YOU CAN TAKE:

Avoid nagging and preaching

Encourage honesty and positive thinking

Promote self-affirmation

Support the process of change

If the person you are caring for has a substance abuse problem, you will probably see the signs. People who abuse drugs or alcohol often deny to themselves, as well as to their loved ones, that they have a problem.

Avoid nagging and preaching

You may want to tell the person with a substance abuse problem what to do. When sincere advice and good suggestions are ignored, you may be tempted to nag and preach to him or her. These are not helpful tactics. If anything, nagging and preaching may make things worse because the person may refuse to listen at all. Try these suggestions instead:

➤ **Let the person know that you are aware of his or her problem.**

Bringing the substance abuse problem "out into the open" is important, particularly since people with substance abuse problems tend to deny that they have a problem. However, be careful to do this *without accusing and judging* the person. Accusations will cause him or her to lie and hide information.

➤ **Suggest getting help from a counselor or support group.**

Encouraging him or her in an honest, straightforward manner to seek professional helps show that you are concerned and that you care. A forceful or nagging approach will not produce the results you desire. Do not make threats to take certain actions unless you fully intend to carry them out. Substance abusers easily learn to ignore suggestions, opinions, and threats unless there are actual consequences.

➤ **Expect setbacks and broken promises, yet be persistent in your concern and caring.**

The life of the person who is chemically dependent is often filled with failures, half-hearted attempts to change, and broken promises. Do not become discouraged if his or her attempts to overcome substance abuse are not successful. Encouraging him or her to try again is far more helpful than preaching about lack of willpower and determination. "Shaming" the person about failure may stop him or her from even trying to succeed.

Encourage honesty and positive thinking

Lies, deceit, denial, and avoidance are common tactics of a person with substance abuse problem; they help him or her to "protect" the problem and to continue the substance abuse. Honesty undermines these devices and brings the truth to light. If a problem exists, owning up to it is an important step in resolving it. Because people with substance abuse problems are used to failure and have had little success in dealing with the problem, *positive thinking* is also a must in overcoming substance abuse.

➤ **Encourage honest efforts and discourage excuses.**

The person with a substance abuse problem usually perceives the causes of the problems to be outside of himself or herself. This leads to excuses and long explanations as to why he or she could not possibly be at fault for anything that is going wrong. Encourage steps toward dealing with his or her addiction. Discourage excuse-making. You may offer to accompany the person to Narcotics Anonymous or some other support group where help can be obtained. Praise any efforts that he or she makes to deal with the substance abuse. Do not accept blaming or excuses.

> ### Encourage facing the problem of substance abuse honestly.

Admitting that one has a substance abuse problem is not easy, and accepting responsibility for dealing with it is harder still. Unless the person with the substance abuse problem is willing to take that responsibility and accept help, little will be accomplished. You can help by repeating, in a clear, nonjudgmental way, that he or she has a substance abuse problem and that, together, you can do something about it.

> ### Encourage positive thinking.

Substance abusers often view life as negative, defeating, discouraging, and failure-ridden. This negative attitude is reinforced by failure—failure to solve the substance abuse problem, for example. If a negative attitude can be replaced with positive suggestions, positive thinking, and positive attitudes, the chances of change and success are greater. An "I can do this" attitude is capable of moving the person, step by step, toward the goal of being drug- or alcohol-free.

Promote self-affirmation

People who battle the problem of substance abuse also battle problems of self-hate, poor self-image, defeatist attitudes, and lack of belief in their own worth. Learning self-respect and how to give and receive love are necessary steps toward a successful and happy life. This is hard work for the person whose love of self and belief in self are often lacking. You, the caregiver, can help by providing him or her with encouragement and affirmation.

> ### Encourage the person to begin to love himself or herself.

Suggest that he or she make a private statement of self-affirmation to himself or herself at the beginning of each day (for example, "I'm really a special person!"). Suggest loving and accepting himself or herself unconditionally. Such love is not selfish, but is wholesome and uplifting.

> ### Demonstrate self-love in your own life.

Demonstrate healthy self-caring by the way you live your own life. Being a role model does not mean preaching. You can demonstrate love for yourself by the choices you make and by the way you treat yourself. This can speak volumes about self-love without saying a word.

> ### Offer positive affirmation.

Giving positive affirmation is letting a person know that you believe that he or she is good and therefore worthy of your love and attention. It also means recognizing the efforts and accomplishments others have made, even if they are small. Compliments, if they are sincere, will bolster morale and self-confidence. Be generous with the affirmations, encouragement, and positive "strokes" that you give.

Support the process of change

Change is often a slow process that requires much effort over a long time. What is truly worth having usually does not come quickly and easily. This is also true of overcoming a substance abuse problem. Change must come one step at a time over a period of weeks, months, or even years. Patience is therefore very important. Expecting too much too soon will only lead to disappointment.

> ### Be patient.

Remember that real change—change that lasts—takes time. If you or the person with a sbustance abuse problem expect too much too soon, you are setting yourself up for disappointment.

> ### Discourage procrastination.

Of course, making changes requires more than good intentions and wishes. It requires that a person act and persist. Putting things off (procrastination) is a common problem among people with substance abuse problems. You should discourage procrastination. Remind the person you are caring for that procrastination will keep him or her from achieving change.

> ### After a change has been accomplished, evaluate the results.

It is important to evaluate what has been given up, what has been accomplished, or what has changed. Changes are never easy, but the results we feel can usually tell us that our decisions were good. The person with a substance abuse problem will *feel* the results: The body usually begins to feel better, and life becomes brighter and more promising. These are signs that the decision to stop drug and alcohol use was a good one.

> ### Aim for changes that are achievable, satisfying, and necessary.

One sure way to fail in any endeavor is to try to accomplish more than is possible. This leads to a cycle of defeat, which, in turn, causes poor self-esteem. Encourage making small changes at first, and then give praise for even these small changes. These small achievements build self-confidence. He or she can then go on to make more difficult changes. Building on small successes is more effective than picking up the pieces after failure to reach a difficult goal.

4. POSSIBLE OBSTACLES TO CAREGIVING

Here are some common attitudes and misconceptions that may prevent you from carrying out your plan:

"I don't *really* have a problem with alcohol or drugs. I can stop using them whenever I choose."

Response: This is a common statement that indicates denial. Perhaps the person with substance abuse has actually convinced himself or herself that this is true. He or she would certainly like *you* to believe this. Without being accusing or judgmental, let him or her know that you see this as sign of denial. Show that you expect honesty and will not "play along" with denial tactics. This will show that *honesty* about the problem will *not* result in preaching and criticism.

Lying, excuse-making, and denial are often a way of life for people with substance abuse problems. Therefore, do not become too discouraged when this behavior occurs.

"Smoking a 'joint' occasionally or popping a pill takes away the anxiety I feel."

Response: This statement could be a trap. Who would not want to see a loved one less anxious or fearful? It is tempting to believe that anything that could spare the person you are caring for from anxiety is acceptable. However, you need to remind yourself that drugs and alcohol do not really help people deal with their anxieties; they merely mask the anxieties for a short time. Once the effects of the chemicals or drugs wear off, the problems and the anxieties will surface once again.

Think of other obstacles

Identify additional roadblocks that could keep you from following the recommendations in this home care plan:

- Will the person I am caring for cooperate?

- Will other people help?

- How can I explain my needs to others?

- Do I have the time and energy to carry out this plan?

You need to develop plans for getting around these roadblocks. Use the four COPE ideas (Creativity, Optimism, Planning, and Expert information) in developing your plans. See pp 4–8 for a discussion of how to use the COPE ideas in overcoming your obstacles.

5. CARRYING OUT AND ADJUSTING YOUR PLAN

Carrying out your plan

A person with a substance abuse problem who also happens to have HIV/AIDS is no different than a person with a substance abuse problem who does *not* have this disease. The goal of treatment for both is a life free of drug and alcohol abuse. It is important to remember that progress is usually slow. Also bear in mind that overcoming drug or alcohol dependency is his or her responsibility, not yours. Success will depend on the desire for change and the effort he or she makes.

What to do if your plan does not work

If honest efforts have been made and the person you love and care about still has the substance abuse problem, it is time to honestly re-evaluate the problem. Re-read the suggestions in this chapter. If there are any suggestions that you have not tried, try them. Of course, a great deal will depend on the willingness of the person with the substance abuse problem. Encourage the person you are caring for to see a counselor, psychiatrist, physician, or clergyman for help. Help can also be obtained from support groups such as Narcotics Anonymous and Alcoholics Anonymous. Be encouraging, supportive, realistic, and persistent. Meanwhile, remember to pay attention to your own needs because living with a person with a substance abuse problem can be very stressful. You might consider attending a support group yourself—for example, Al-Anon, a support group for those whose lives are affected by people with alcohol abuse problems.

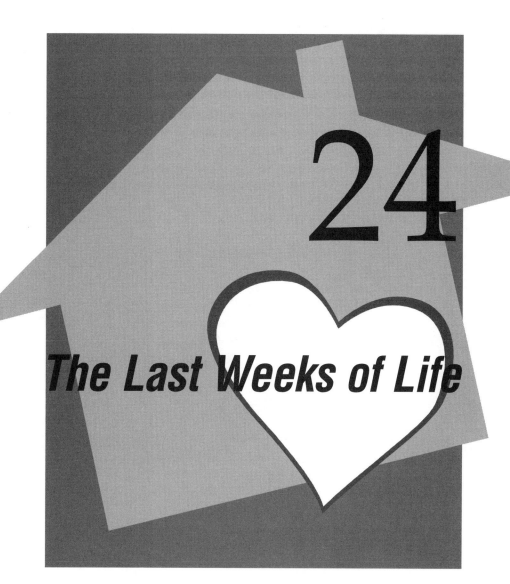

24

The Last Weeks of Life

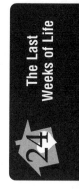

Overview of the Home Care Plan for
The Last Weeks of Life

 1. UNDERSTANDING THE PROBLEM

        Sharing fears regarding death

        Planning care for the terminal phase of the illness

        Discussing plans for the time of death

        Your goals

 2. WHEN TO GET PROFESSIONAL HELP

        Understanding what calling 911 means

        When to call for professional help

 3. WHAT YOU CAN DO TO HELP

        Provide comfort and rest

        Welcome visitors

        Other special concerns during the last weeks of life

 4. POSSIBLE OBSTACLES TO CAREGIVING

5. CARRYING OUT AND ADJUSTING YOUR PLAN

        Carrying out your plan

        What to do if your plan does not work

> **Topics that have an arrow (➤) in front of them are actions you can take or symptoms you can look for.**

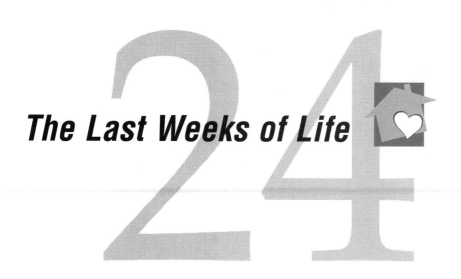

The Last Weeks of Life

1. UNDERSTANDING THE PROBLEM

Any book that discusses common problems of persons with HIV/AIDS would not be complete without a discussion of the issue of death. All persons who face a serious illness such as advanced cancer or AIDS are forced to think about death.

Not all persons with HIV/AIDS will die of their disease—but many will. When the disease is progressing, it is important to think about and plan for death because it is a possibility. The person with HIV/AIDS should be encouraged to talk openly about how he or she would like to die and what wishes he or she would like honored after death. Having a trusted friend, loved one, counselor, or clergyperson

> ➤ The information in this home care plan fits most situations, but yours may be different.
>
> ➤ If the doctor or nurse tells you to do something else, follow what he or she says.
>
> ➤ If you think there may be a medical emergency, see the section "When To Get Professional Help" on pp 288–292.

with whom to share fears and concerns about death can be very helpful. Unfortunately, the person with HIV/AIDS and those closest to him or her often hide their thoughts and feelings about death to avoid upsetting each other, and pretend that such feelings do not even exist. As a result, these issues are never properly discussed; the person with HIV/AIDS does not get the kind of care he or she wants just before death, and his or her wishes are not carried out *after* death. If you, the caregiver, have questions or concerns about these issues, you can start a conversation by sharing what you feel. This may open the door for the person with HIV/AIDS to discuss his or her feelings as well.

It is helpful to explore with the person with HIV/AIDS his or her wishes regarding the extent of treatment he or she would like to receive. Some people feel that they would simply like to be kept comfortable as they approach death and would not want to receive "heroic measures" that will merely keep them alive or that would deprive them of quality of life. Others feel that they would want everything done to help them live longer. *Knowing the wishes of the person with HIV/AIDS is very important.* Those wishes can be formally documented in the Living Will and Durable Power of Attorney forms. These forms are designed to express clearly personal desires for treatment during the period of terminal illness just before death.

If the person with HIV/AIDS has young children, arrangements must be made for their care, including the appointment of a legal guardian.

The person with HIV/AIDS must make a will, choose the person who is to be the power of attorney for finance and the person who is to be the durable power of attorney for medical decisions (the person who will make medical decisions when the person with HIV/AIDS is no longer able to do so). Funeral arrangements should also be discussed early. This will ensure that the wishes of the person with HIV/AIDS will be honored. Signing a Living Will and selecting a durable power of attorney is referred to as signing "Advance Directives." Talking about Advance Directives can be difficult. Patients must openly confront the seriousness of their condition, and decisions about what to do and who to include at the end of life can be emotionally stressful. Doctors, nurses, social workers, or hospice volunteers can help.

YOUR GOALS

Know when to get professional help

Provide comfort and rest

Welcome visitors

2. ***WHEN TO GET PROFESSIONAL HELP***

➤ **Understand what calling 911 means.**

When you call 911 or the number of the emergency response team in your area, bear in mind that the ambulance team will arrive expecting to save a life or to give "aggressive treatment"—even if, in most states, the person has a living will containing wishes to the contrary. Ambulance crews are required by law to do this. Aggressive treatment means inserting tubes, performing CPR (cardiopulmonary resuscitation) if the heart has stopped beating, and resuscitating the person if he or she has stopped breathing. These attempts to restore life rarely work for persons with late-stage HIV/AIDS, and they do not help with comfort.

It may take time to persuade the ambulance crew that you want help controlling a symptom such as difficulty breathing or pain and that you do not necessarily want them to save a life. Any emergency team will want to know who the primary doctor is, and they may want to call him or her after the situation is "under control"—that is, after the distressing symptom has been relieved. If the person with AIDS is close to death, expect the emergency team to do what they know best: life-saving action. They will also probably move the patient from the home to the hospital and even admit them to an intensive care unit.

Once he or she is in a hospital, whatever is in a living will may be ignored until the physicians agree that he or she can be allowed to die a natural death. In many states, a living will that is valid at home is not valid at a hospital until a doctor puts it in the hospital chart. Sometimes living wills that were put in the chart earlier are lost. In this case, you will need to obtain a new one. Do not assume that a living will that was accepted in one hospital will automatically be accepted at other hospitals.

Some small towns, rural areas, and certain states allow communication between home health agencies and hospices and local 911 or emergency response teams to prevent these problems. If the patient and family agree, hospice staff can inform local emergency teams in advance about who has a terminal illness and what the goals of the emergency team should be if anyone calls for "emergency" help. Unfortunately, many states do not permit this type of practical information exchange and do not let 911 teams follow the wishes of a living will. Check to see what is allowed in your area by asking your hospice team.

➤ **Let all those who are assisting with caregiving know when they should and should not call 911.**

Be sure to tell others who are helping with caregiving—such as those people who "sit" with the person with HIV/AIDS or those that provide nursing care—under what circumstances they should call 911. If the person you are caring for does *not wish* to receive any aggressive life-saving measures from an ambulance team, let other caregivers know that they should *not* call 911—but *should* call the visiting nurse, hospice, or doctor's office. Post this information on the refrigerator or near the phone to remind other caregivers of these wishes when you are not at home.

If the person *does wish* to receive aggressive life-saving measures, then it is appropriate to call 911. *Do* call the ambulance crew or emergency response team if the person you are caring for has fallen, is in pain, or is choking.

If you are in doubt as to whether or not you should call 911, call the hospice or home health staff who are helping you. They can decide what step is best to take next, and they are available 24 hours a day.

Call for professional help if any of the following occurs:

➤ **The person you are caring for is experiencing severe pain.**

There is no reason that a person who is close to death should be in pain. Medicines for pain control, anxiety, and the relief of other unpleasant symptoms should be given as long as the person is alive. However, the way that these medicines are taken may need to be changed. For example, if it is hard for the person to swallow medicines, they can be prescribed in the form of injections, suppositories, or even skin "patches." Call the doctor and ask for these changes. Pain that is not controlled may need to be carefully monitored, with adjustments being made to the pain medication. Sometimes the person with HIV/AIDS may need to be hospitalized for a short period to accomplish proper pain control. See the home care plan "Pain" (Chapter 14) for more information about pain control.

➤ **The person you are caring for is having trouble breathing.**

It is very difficult to watch someone you love struggle to breathe. This experience can cause you and the person with HIV/AIDS to become frightened and anxious. Sometimes shortness of breath occurs during the last weeks of life because of weakness, anemia (low count of red blood cells, which carry oxygen in the blood), or the presence of disease in the lungs. Health professionals can do things to relieve or reduce this problem.

> ### The person is confused or is experiencing hallucinations.

Confusion or hallucinations can be caused by AIDS dementia complex (ADC; see the home care plan "AIDS Dementia Complex,"Chapter 15). It can also be caused by narcotic overdoses or by natural processes that occur during the process of dying. Whatever the reason, people who are experiencing severe confusion may not know where they are or who they are with. This is not a real problem during the last weeks or days of life unless the person you are caring for is unhappy about where he or she thinks he is. It might make him or her cry or be afraid or see things that are not there. Sometimes these visions are of people who have already died, such as a mother or a child. These are called hallucinations—seeing things that are not there. If the visions are comforting, however, hallucinations are not a problem during the last days of life. They are a problem only if the hallucinations are frightening or upsetting. Call for professional help if this is the case.

> ### The person you are caring is experiencing prolonged or severe anxiety.

Sometimes anxiety is caused by medicines. If so, the doctor may order a different medicine or prescribe anti-anxiety medicine. Other times, anxiety can come from feeling disoriented or not in control. For example, a person might feel like he or she is falling off a chair even though he or she is flat in a hospital bed. Whatever the reason, try to understand what is frightening the person you are caring for. Do not make assumptions: You could be wrong, which would hinder your ability to help. It is OK to ask the person what worries him or her the most. This allows you to focus on the real issues, rather than guessing at what the person is afraid of. For example, you may assume the person is afraid of dying when, in reality, he or she is afraid of being left alone or is afraid of using up his or her money. See the home care plan "Coping with Anxiety" (Chapter 18) for suggestions on how to help alleviate anxiety.

> ### The person you are caring for has fallen and you believe he or she may be injured.

Toward the end of life, people become very weak and are at much higher risk of falling when walking or sitting. If you are alone, you may be unable to help the person up from the floor. Even if you are able to help the person to a chair, you may feel that the fall was a serious one and that medical assistance is necessary. In either case, **call 911 immediately** for emergency assistance. Members of the ambulance squad can help the person up from the floor, and are trained to look for injuries such as broken bones or head injury. This will determine the need for a trip to the hospital.

➤ **You feel that you cannot go on caring for the person with HIV/AIDS at home because the care has become too difficult.**

It is not unusual for caregivers of persons who are very ill to become overwhelmed by the responsibilities involved. Physicians, nurses, and social workers who care for HIV/AIDS patients can help you decide if you can continue to provide care in the home and how to get some days of respite care in a hospital or nursing facility for the person with HIV/AIDS while you get some rest and relief. Nursing home care or care at a palliative care unit or in-patient hospice are other options. With these alternatives, you can still visit and help as a family member, but are not responsible 24 hours a day. See the home care plan "Getting Help from Community Agencies and Volunteer Groups" (Chapter 21) for more information on whom to contact for professional help for this problem.

➤ **People in the household are scared by the thought of having the person with HIV/AIDS die at home.**

The caregiver, the person with HIV/AIDS, and others who may be living in the home may become frightened by the idea of death within the home. They may be worried about what to do if unexpected difficulties arise. Being honest about these concerns and discussing them with a doctor, nurse, or social worker will often reduce these fears and feelings of helplessness.

WHAT YOU CAN DO TO HELP

If the decision has been made to keep the person with HIV/AIDS at home as the time of death slowly gets closer, here are some goals you can strive to meet.

Provide comfort and rest

Rest and sleep are very important during the terminal phase of the illness. You may notice that the person you are caring for wants to sleep more. The body is worn out not only from fighting the disease but also from the difficult treatments. Getting the sleep he or she needs will help the person with HIV/AIDS to feel more refreshed and to have some quality time when awake.

➤ **Give medicines for pain and discomfort on a regular basis.**

Strive to keep the person as comfortable as possible. Many people feel that once the sick person is asleep, he or she will feel no pain. This is not always true. Pain can be felt during sleep and may prevent the person from getting a restful sleep. Continue to give pain medication at night if pain has been a problem. A good way to judge if pain is controlled during sleep is to pay attention to whether the person is waking up with a great deal of pain. If so, this means that the pain medicine has worn off and probably should be given more often. You should talk to the doctor about changing the type of pain medication used or the intervals between doses. Another important part of pain control is to give medicines before the pain builds up—on a regular time schedule, so that the blood levels of the medicine are always high enough to control the pain. See the home care plan "Pain" (Chapter 14) for more information about controlling pain.

➤ Play soft, relaxing music and use dim lighting.

Music can be very soothing to the spirit. Some people use music with meditation or relaxation techniques to relax. Because people who are ill are often bothered by bright lights and may even develop headaches from them, use dim lighting in your home. Soft lighting, especially when accompanied by soft, gentle music, can create an atmosphere of relaxation and peace.

➤ Help the person you are caring for remain comfortable in bed.

Lying in the same position hour after hour can cause the joints and muscles to become stiff and sore and can also lead to pressure sores and skin breakdown. Help the person you are caring for to change position every 2 to 4 hours, if this is comfortable for him or her. Placing a folded sheet under the midsection of the body allows two people to turn the person or to move him or her up in the bed without discomfort, tugging, or pulling on limbs. Massaging hands, feet, and the back will help prevent skin sores and increase comfort.

➤ Prevent bedsores.

Sometimes, despite your best efforts to help him or her change position in bed several times a day, bedsores will develop because of constant pressure against the skin. Bedsores start under the skin, and you may not know that they are present until they become severe. At first, bedsore will appear pink; they then change to red, the skin opens up, and the size of the sore increases quickly. They are often painful. They are most likely to occur at places on the body that are "bony": the ankles, heels, tailbone, hips, and elbows. See the home care plan "Skin Problems" (Chapter 11), pp 127–128, for further suggestions on preventing bedsores. Call for professional help if you notice very red areas on the skin or open sores.

➤ Provide back rubs and skin care using a pleasant lotion or cream.

Back rubs and skin massages are comforting and enjoyable to most people. Most people feel loved when they are touched in a gentle, caring way. Using lotions or creams to massage the skin (during the shorter massage—*i.e., less than 1 minute*) will keep it from getting too dry, will promote circulation, and will prevent cracks and sore areas. Avoid using lotions that contain alcohol, because alcohol dries the skin.

➤ Use a pan for bathing.

If the person you are caring for is unable to get in the bathtub or shower anymore, he or she can sit on the toilet seat or on a chair in front of the sink and use a pan to bathe himself or herself. If the person is too weak to do even this, you can assist with bathing by washing him or her from the pan. If the person does not want to get out of bed, you can sponge-bathe him or her in the bed. During bathing, be sure to keep the person covered with a soft sheet or blanket to avoid a chill as well as to give privacy. Start with the face, then wash the arms and legs, the chest and back, and finally, the private area. A nurse's aide or nurse can help you with bathing, if necessary.

➤ Consider using an electric hospital bed.

Electric beds are easy to operate. The person with HIV/AIDS and you are able to control positions on your own. Hospital beds are also available that are nonelectric. A crank at the bottom is used to raise the bed up and down and to elevate the head or feet. However, cranking is more difficult to do and requires that someone bend to operate the crank. The bed can be kept in the living room or den on the first floor to make it easier for the caregiver and so that visitors have more room to visit. Hospital beds can be ordered by any visiting nurses or can be obtained by calling a durable medical equipment supply store (see the Yellow Pages of the phone book), which will deliver it and set it up. The cost of rental is usually covered by insurance.

➤ Continue to let the person you are caring for plan the day.

Letting the person you are caring for plan his or her day is a way of showing respect and support. Let the person you are caring for plan what to do, what to eat or drink, when to sleep, when to watch television, and when to visit with others.

➤ Touch and talk.

Even if the person you are caring for is sleeping much of the time or slips into a coma, touching and talking remain important. Touch can include back rubs or hand-holding. Visitors can read scriptures or stories, talk about old times, or read poems. Background music may also help. All of these decrease the sense of being alone and can be very comforting.

➤ Keep the lips and mouth clean and moist.

People who are terminally ill eat and drink less. This leads to a dry mouth and cracked, sore lips. Encourage and remind the person you are caring for to clean the teeth and to rinse the mouth at least several times each day, so that the mouth feels comfortable. Lip balm or ointment will keep the lips from drying and cracking.

➤ Use the end of a straw to help the person take small sips of liquids.

During the last weeks of life, some people are too weak to drink from a glass. In this case, you can help give fluids using a straw. First, dip the straw into the glass and hold your finger over the end of the straw. This will hold liquid in the straw. You can then drip the liquid into the person's mouth by releasing the finger quickly and then covering it again. Fill the straw with only a very small amount of liquid, to avoid releasing too much into the mouth of the person who is ill. Practice this before actually trying to give liquids this way.

➤ Use a special spoon to give liquid medicines.

Pharmacies carry special medicine spoons that help prevent spilling liquid medicine. The spoon handle is enclosed and looks like a tube. You can pour the medicine into the scoop part, and it will flow down into the tube into the mouth. It is much easier to take medicine such as Maalox with this type of spoon. You might also trying giving medicines with a syringe. Have a nurse show you how to use it. If the person you are caring for is having trouble swallowing, placing a few drops under the tongue will still allow the medicine to be absorbed.

➤ Ease discomfort caused by fever.

Sometimes fevers develop because not enough liquid is taken. In this case, encourage the person you are caring for to drink more. Cool cloths applied to the brow are also helpful. Do not give icy or cold baths. In some cases, the doctor may order antibiotics if the person you are caring for has an infection. (For a more detailed discussion of fever and infection, see the home care plan "Fever and Infections" [Chapter 5].)

➤ Manage and prevent problems with bleeding.

Sometimes bumping the arms or wrists (against furniture, for example) during everyday movements can cause minor skin bleeding in the person with HIV/AIDS during the advanced stages of the disease. This is because the skin is not as tough as it once was. Medicines may also bring about changes in skin, causing it to be easily scraped open. Small gauze pads can be placed over any open spots and wrapped with 1-or 2-inch gauze to stay in place. Avoid using tape, as this may tear the skin open.

If a nosebleed occurs, tilt the head back, but do not have the person lie flat. Lying flat might make him or her choke on blood dripping from the nose into the throat. Put ice wrapped in a washcloth on the nose for short periods (2 minutes). Applying pressure to the skin and nose stops most bleeding. However, internal bleeding or bleeding that causes blood to appear in the urine or stool cannot be stopped in this way because you cannot apply pressure to these areas. If bleeding from the nose or other places continues, call the visiting nurse. The physician may order medications to slow down the bleeding.

➤ Soak feet in warm water.

Many people enjoy the feeling of warm water and miss bathing in a shower or tub. You can make up for this by helping the person soak his or her feet in a pan of warm water. Do one foot at a time, allowing each foot to soak for about 10 minutes.

➤ Change sheets at least twice a week.

If the person you are caring for is spending more time in bed, the sheets will get soiled more quickly. The feeling of fresh sheets is comforting, so change the sheets at least twice a week. If the person spends a great deal of time resting on a sofa or recliner chair, a fresh sheet cover should be placed on these places, too.

Welcome visitors

Not everyone is comfortable visiting a person who is approaching death. Some people want to stay away, and others want to come and offer help. During the last weeks of life, the person you are caring for should continue to have control over whom to see and visit with. Here are some ideas to help you manage visitors at this time:

➤ Set special visiting hours.

You and the person you are caring for should decide which hours of the day should be set aside for visitors. Otherwise, visitors may come and go all day, and you may find it hard to turn them away. Tell people the "visiting hours" ahead of time, and stick to this schedule. This way, you and the person you are caring for will have time for rest and personal care.

➤ Invite your clergyman or support group members to visit.

Prayers and conversations with a clergyman or with fellow support group members can be very comforting during the last weeks of life for some people. Priests or deacons may want to bring sacraments such as communion. Many home health agencies and hospice groups have a chaplain on staff who can also visit. These visits should not be forced. It is up to the person with HIV/AIDS to decide whom he or she is comfortable talking with.

> ### Tell visitors if they are staying too long.

Let visitors know ahead of time how long a visit should last. If the person you are caring for becomes tired sooner than you anticipated, however, let visitors know. At this stage of the illness, most people will appreciate your honesty, and will want to know if they are staying too long. If the person you are caring for is too weak to see people, ask if he or she would like to try "visits" over the telephone instead.

> ### Allow the person you are caring for to decide whom he or she will visit.

The person you are caring for has the right to decide whom he or she will visit, especially during the last weeks of life. He or she may not want to see certain people, or, if it is a bad day, anyone at all. Ask the person whom he or she wants to see, and then invite them.

Anticipate and prepare for problems

Families usually prepare carefully when they expect the birth of a baby. However, many families avoid planning when helping someone through the last days of life. As a result, friends and loved ones often do not know what to expect or what to do when death is close. Be prepared by taking the following steps:

> ### Keep phone numbers of home health nurses, hospice nurses, and doctors in a convenient place.

Having phone numbers ready will help in a time of crisis or immediate need. If the person you are caring for has a sudden emergency, you will want to reach a health care professional quickly. Keep important phone numbers in a place where you and others can reach them easily.

> ### Keep a sufficient supply of needed medicines (for example, pain medications, anti-nausea medicines, and anti-anxiety medications) in the home for emergencies.

You do not want to deal with phone calls for prescriptions and trips to the pharmacy to pick up medicines when the person you are caring for needs them immediately. One of the most frightening experiences for a person who is ill is to have symptoms arise and not have the necessary medications available. This may cause you to panic, too. Keep prescriptions filled, and check with your pharmacy to be sure that they keep a supply of these medicines.

➤ **Keep a written list of the instructions you receive from doctors or nurses.**

Keep a special notebook or folder that is used only for writing down the instructions that doctors and nurses give you. Most important are instructions on which problems to watch for or anticipate and on what to do if these problems arise. During an emergency, you will not want to waste time searching for instructions. Keeping instructions in a special notebook and keeping this notebook close at hand will help you act quickly and decisively during an emergency.

➤ **Arrange in advance for family, friends, or volunteers to help you with caregiving.**

During the terminal stage of the disease, being the only caregiver is almost impossible and very stressful. Make arrangements ahead of time to have others help you with caregiving. If you do not know whom to ask, let the nurse or social worker who is working with you know that you need help at home.

➤ **Locate bills, checks, records of accounts, and important papers such as insurance policies.**

The person you are caring for may have shared decision-making with you about finances and accounts. If not, it is time to locate important papers about finances and accounts. Find out what the papers mean and what needs to be done with them to put accounts in order.

➤ **Ask the bank ahead of time how accounts are handled after someone dies.**

The bank will probably tell you that the bank account must be in both your name and the name of the other person for you to be able to withdraw funds after that person dies. If the account is not in both your names, put both your names on the account *before* the person dies.

➤ **Learn new household chores.**

If the person you are caring for has always been responsible for certain household chores in the past, such as shopping, preparing meals, or cleaning clothes, you will need to learn to do them yourself or you will need to ask someone to do them for you. Nurses' aides and home helpers can do some shopping and run errands, but they may not visit every day and do not always have time to do these chores. If you cannot do these chores yourself, it is usually better to ask friends, neighbors, or relatives to help.

➤ **Talk with a friend about your feelings.**

Being with a close friend or someone you can talk to is an excellent way to sort out your feelings. Knowing that others care and are there to listen is reassuring. Friends can give you the support, strength, and confidence you need to get through during this difficult experience.

➤ **Plan something nice for yourself at least once a day.**

Many caregivers make the mistake of not taking any time for themselves and of feeling guilty if they do. Now more than ever you need to plan pleasant activities for yourself. These activities could be as simple as going to lunch with a friend or taking a nap. The home care plan "Creating and Maintaining Positive Experiences" (Chapter 19) offers several ideas on pleasant activities you can try.

Other special concerns during the last weeks of life

If you and the person you are caring for have decided that he or she will stay at home during the last weeks of life, there are some special concerns that you will need to consider:

1. What should be done in the event of a medical problem.

   Because comfort is the primary goal of care for a dying patient, your doctor may suggest little or no medical treatment for problems if the treatment makes the patient uncomfortable. Another difficult question is whether or not the person you are caring for should enter a hospital. These are not issues you should try to resolve on your own. Discuss them with your doctor.

2. What hospice services are available.

   Hospice is a service for dying patients and family members who take care of these patients at home. Nurses and social workers make house calls and help family caregivers find ways to keep the patient comfortable. They may also assist in getting extra help to care for the patient at home. Sometimes dying patients go to residential hospice units where they may stay for weeks or months. Both home and residential hospice staff are skilled in relieving pain and shortness of breath for dying patients.

3. What should be done just before the person you are caring for dies.

Usually it is clear when death is near because the patient with HIV/AIDS sleeps most of the time, eats and drinks very little, and may breathe differently.

➤ Understand when to call 911 and when *not* to call.

Sometimes, when family caregivers see that the person with HIV/AIDS is going to die soon, they are tempted to call an ambulance. *Instead of calling 911, call the hospice nurse, visiting nurse, or doctor and explain that the person you are caring for is going to die soon.* They will advise you on what to do.

➤ Do not feel guilty about being unable to "do enough."

You may find yourself worrying that you are not doing enough to help the person you are caring for to feel better. Do not feel guilty about this. Nothing you do or don't do will change what is happening. You really won't make any "wrong" decisions about the care of the person with HIV/AIDS. The important point is to remember to keep the person as comfortable as possible, without worrying that you are not doing "enough" to provide comfort.

➤ Find out who wants to visit near the time of death to say final good-byes.

After you decide, with the help of family and close friends, who should be informed of the person's death, make a list of their names with their phone numbers. However, not everyone will be home or available by phone when you first try to reach them. You might then ask someone else to take responsibility for calling the people who could not be reached the first time.

➤ Decide who would be most helpful to you near the time of death.

You are likely to feel tired and "stressed" at this time. This is when you need and should *receive* help.

Knowing ahead of time what to do when the person you are caring for dies will help you deal with this very difficult experience. Write down your plan and keep it handy.

➤ Do not feel you need to call the funeral home immediately after the person dies.

After the person you are caring for dies, the hospice nurse might be the first person you call. A death certificate must be completed and funeral arrangements made, but these things do not need to be done right away. Family members and loved ones may want to visit the bedside of the patient and grieve before the funeral home staff members come.

After the death, some people want to "get on with it" and have the body picked up quickly by the funeral home. Other people prefer to sit with the body, cry, and talk. Sometimes friends and family who were not present at death want to see the body before it is moved from the last place that the person was. If this is important, wait for the others to arrive and express their grief. Time is no longer a pressure. The body can stay in the home for quite some time before funeral staff needs to pick it up. If the person died in a chair, it is best to lie the body on a couch or bed after death and after the first good-byes are said. Even if the person has lost a lot of weight, lifting the body will be difficult. It will probably take at least two adults to move the body.

> **Help young children deal with grief.**

Many people with HIV/AIDS have young children, as do their family and friends. The children need to be included in the grieving. Although they may not understand everything, explain as much as you can about what is happening and about the loss that has just taken place. Talking to children about death *before* a person dies can also be helpful. Do not be afraid to show the children that you are sad or upset. Explain the reasons for your emotions.

4. POSSIBLE OBSTACLES TO CAREGIVING

Think about attitudes that could prevent you from carrying out your plans.

Here are some common attitudes and misconceptions that may prevent you from carrying out your plan:

"We have to do everything we can to let him or her live longer."

Response: If the person you are caring for asks that nothing be done to lengthen life (that is, that no "heroic measures" be taken), then this wish must be respected. Remind yourself that it is the quality or comfort of life that is important—not the quantity or length of life.

Usually when people say, "We must do all we can," they are also saying, "I'm not ready to see this person die." They are saving the person's life to prevent themselves from facing his or her death and loss. The only time that heroic measures are appropriate is when the person with HIV/AIDS wants them. Doctors and nurses, as well as loved ones, should talk to the person who is terminally ill *well in advance*

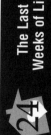

of a crisis or emergency to find out what he or she desires at the end of life.

"If I prepare in advance, people will think that I want her to die."

Response:	Some people will always have their own opinions, no matter what you do. Their thoughts should not determine what you do. What is important are the wishes of the person who will die. Your goal is to respect those wishes, and to do this you must make plans. If you do this, then at the time of death there will be less tension because decisions were thought about and made earlier.

"I don't want the children to remember their uncle like this."

Response:	Seeing very sick persons can be upsetting to children. If you want the children to see their sick relative, you can make it less upsetting by preparing them for what they are going to see. Children are capable of understanding when a person is very ill, but they need someone to give them information in a manner that they can understand. They also need someone with whom they can talk about their feelings and someone who will answer their questions.

5. CARRYING OUT AND ADJUSTING YOUR PLAN

Carrying out your plan

As the end of life approaches, many decisions need to be made. This time can be very stressful. It is hoped that you as the caregiver have other people to help. Many of the ideas in this home care plan can be carried out by friends or caring others who are willing to assist you. Help from home health nurses and hospice staff is available as well. Ask others to do those things that you cannot get to or to help you with difficult tasks or decisions that you would rather not handle alone. People are usually willing to help. Most of the time they are just waiting to be asked.

What to do if your plan does not work

Helping someone to die at home can be difficult, but it can also be a very rewarding experience. This is because you have respected the wishes of the person who wants to die at home. However, if you need to take the person with HIV/AIDS to a residential hospice unit to live out the last days of life, you have not failed as a caregiver. You have tried your best, and that is all that anyone can ask of you. Remember that you have choices. If caring for the person at home is not working out as planned, discuss the matter honestly. You and the person you are caring for should try to come up with a plan that is acceptable to both of you. The important thing is that you both talk about the process of dying and prepare for it in a way that is helpful for both of you.

Appendices

Appendix A:
Helpful Resources and
Phone Numbers

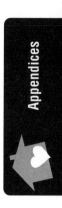

State and National Agencies

➤ **The American Foundation for AIDS Research (AMFAR).** This agency supports clinical research projects, provides community education, and publishes a treatment directory. Telephone: **(212) 333-3118** or **(213) 273-5547.**

➤ **The Centers for Disease Control and Prevention—AIDS Activity Project.** This agency offers educational materials, a listing of HIV testing sites, and national reports on the disease of AIDS. Telephone: **(404) 639-2891.**

➤ **The Fund for Human Dignity.** This agency offers counseling and referral information (A National Directory of AIDS-Related Services and AIDS Service Agencies). Telephone: **(212) 529-1600** or **1-800-221-7044** (crisis line).

➤ **Gay Men's Health Crisis.** This agency offers legal aid, financial aid, housing, counseling, and educational information. Telephone: **(212) 807-6655.**

Local Support Services

➤ **DC AIDS Task Force.** This service offers counseling, support groups, an IV drug program, legal aid, transportation, and more. Telephone: **(202) 332-5295** or **(202) 332-EXAM** (HIV testing line).

➤ **AIDS Institute of New York.** This service offers housing, community education, legal aid, counseling, and HIV testing sites information. Telephone: **(212) 340-3388.**

➤ **Seattle AIDS Action Project.** This service offers AIDS testing, counseling, support groups, and direct service referrals. Telephone: **(206) 323-1229.**

➤ **PWA (People With AIDS) Coalition in New York City.** This service offers community education, support groups for AIDS patients and women with AIDS, experimental treatment information, and the handbook "Striving and Thriving with AIDS." Telephone: **(212) 566-4995.**

➤ **AIDS Services of Chicago.** This service offers counseling; support groups for patients, others, and the worried well; buddies; testing for HIV; legal referrals; and speakers on the topic of AIDS. Telephone: **(312) 871-5777.**

➤ **Baltimore Health Education Resource Organization (HERO).** This service offers community and professional education, support groups, buddies, housing, transportation, prison outreach, minority outreach, and financial help. Telephone: **(410) 945-AIDS.**

➤ **Philadelphia AIDS Task Force.** This service offers housing for PWAs, HIV testing and counseling, education, and medical and dental referrals. Telephone: **(215) 545-8686.**

➤ **AIDS Foundation of Houston.** This service offers a buddy program, counseling on legal affairs, support groups for PWAs and health care workers, food and clothing bank, physician referral, financial assistance, rent assistance, and transportation. Telephone: **(713) 623-6796.**

Other helpful resources

➤ "A Guide to Home Care for the Person with AIDS." A 31-page illustrated booklet with advice for both people with AIDS and their caregivers. Contact your local chapter of the American Red Cross, and ask for form #329542.

➤ Free pamphlets such as "Preventing HIV/AIDS" (#D-712), "Caring for Someone with AIDS" (#D-498) and the new Surgeon General's Report on Aids (#D-323). Call the National AIDS Clearinghouse at **1-800-458-5231.**

➤ Answers to questions, free written materials, and referrals to local services; 24-hours-a-day, confidential:

• National AIDS Hotline of the U.S. Centers for Disease Control and Prevention: **1-800-342-AIDS.**

• Spanish language hotline: **1-800-344-7432.**

• TTY hotline for the hearing impaired: **1-800-243-7432.**

• Project Inform: **1-800-822-7422.**

• National Institute of Drug Abuse Hotline: **1-800-662-HELP.**

• National Sexually Transmitted Disease Hotline: **1-800-227-8922.**

• National Child Abuse Hotline: **1-800-422-4453.**

• AIDS Information Network: **(215) 575-1110.**

➤ Information on pastoral counseling and support services, The AIDS National Interfaith Network at **1-800-288-9619.**

➤ Family HIV/AIDS Support Helpline operated by Parents, Families, and Friends of Lesbians and Gays. Information on local groups. Telephone: **(202) 638-4200.**

➤ "AIDS and Aging—What People Over 50 Need to Know," program for small-group discussion. Contact HealthCare Education Associates: **(714) 240-2179.**

➤ Fact sheet on AIDS and older adults from the National Institutes on Aging. Telephone: **1-800-222-2225.**

➤ AARP fact sheet. "AIDS: A Multigenerational Crisis" stock no. D14942. Write AARP/SOS, Dept. B, 601 E Street, NW, Washington, D.C. 20049. Includes referral sources for finding help.

Appendix B: Helpful Resources and Phone Numbers in Canada

➤ Canadian AIDS Society, 400-100 Sparks Street, Ottawa, Ontario K1P5B7. Telephone: **(613) 230-3580.**

➤ AIDS Committee of Ottawa, 207 Queen Street, 4th Floor, Ottawa, Ontario K1P6E5. Telephone: **(613) 238-5014.**

➤ AIDS Committee of Toronto, 399 Church Street, Toronto, Ontario M5B2J6. Telephone: **(416) 340-2437.**

➤ AIDS New Brunswick, 65 Brunswick Street, Frederickton, New Brunswick E3B1G5. Telephone: **(506) 450-2782.**

➤ AIDS Prince Rupert, Box 848, Prince Rupert, British Columbia V8J3Y1. Telephone: **(604) 627-8823.**

➤ AIDS Vancouver, Pacific AIDS Resources Center, 1107 Seymour Street, Vancouver, British Columbia V6B558. Telephone: **(604) 681-2122.**

Appendix C:
Medicines Used in the Treatment of HIV Infection

Name	Trade Name	Uses	Possible Side Effects	Comments	Interactions
Acyclovir	Zovirax	Used to treat herpes infections	Few		
Dapsone	—	Used to prevent *pneumocystis carinii* pneumonia	Decreased red blood counts; also alters liver function		Decreased dapsone level if the patient is also taking rifampin
Didanosine (ddl)	Videx	Fights HIV by decreasing the amount of virus produced	Numbness, tingling or pain in toes and fingertips; abdominal pain from inflammation of the pancreas (pancreatitis); diarrhea		
Ethambutol	Myambutol	Used to treat MAC	Can affect red-green vision		
Fluconazole	Diflucan	For yeast infections, such as oral thrush or vaginal infections			
Ganciclovir	—	Used to treat CMV infections such as retinitis (infection of the retina)	Decreased white blood cell counts, blood calcium and potassium levels	Given intravenously (IV)	
Itraconazole	Sporanox	Used to treat fungus	Nausea, occasionally abdominal pain		Will not be absorbed if used with antacid medications (e.g., Mylanta, Maalox, Zantac, Pepcid)
Isoniazid	Nydrazid Laniazid	Used to treat tuberculosis	Numbness and tingling of fingertips and toes; also affects liver function	Can cause flushing of the face if the patient eats Swiss cheese	May increase the levels of other medicines taken for seizures
Megestrol acetate	Megace	Used to increase appetite	Nausea, vomiting, hair loss, blood clots		
Clotrimazole	Mycelex	Few side effects			
Pentamidine Isethionate	Pentam	Used as inhaler or injected into a vein to prevent or treat *Pneumocystis carinii* pneumonia	Low blood sugar or low blood pressure; when inhaled, can cause wheezing; inhaled form can irritate eyes		
Rifabutin	Mycobutin	Used to prevent MAC, a bacterialike tuberculosis	Orange-brown color of urine, feces, salvia; may stain contact lenses		Decreases the amount of zidovudine in the blood

MAC = mycobacterium avium complex; CMV = cytomegalovirus.

Continued

Medicines Used in the Treatment of HIV Infection—cont'd.

Name	Trade Name	Uses	Side Effects	Comments	Interactions
Rifampin	Rifadin Rimactane	Used to treat tuberculosis	Nausea, fevers, rash		Changes the blood levels of many other drugs
Stavudine (d4T)	Zerit	Fights HIV by decreasing amount of virus made			
Trimethoprim/ sulfamethoxa- zole	Bactrim Septra	Fights bacteria; prevents some HIV-related pneu- monias (*Pneumocystis carinii* pneumonia); also used for bladder infec- tions	Itchy rash (most common side effect); fever; de- creased white blood cell counts	Large pills may be hard to swallow	
Zalcitibine (ddC)	Hivid	Fights HIV by decreasing amount of virus pro- duced	Numbness, tingling, and pain in toes and finger- tips; abdominal pain from inflammation of the pancreas (pancreatitis); painful ulcer in the esophagus (swallowing tube)		
Zidovudine	Retrovir	Fights HIV by decreasing amount of virus pro- duced	Decreased red blood cell counts, nausea, head- ache, loss of appetite, lack of energy		

MAC = mycobacterium avium complex.

Appendix D:
Opportunistic Infections Complicating Late-Stage HIV Infection

Infection (listed alphabetically)	Condition (usual name[s])	Usual Clinical Manifestation(s)
Bacteria		
Bartonella species	Bacillary angiomatosis	Widespread infection (skin, bones, lymph organs and
	Disseminated cat scratch disease	bloodstream)
Haemophilus influenzae	Bacterial pneumonia	Pneumonia
Salmonella species	Salmonellosis	Diarrhea (intestinal infection) or bloodstream
		infection
Shigella species	Bacillary dysentery	Diarrhea (intestinal infection) or bloodstream
		infection
Staphylococcus aureus	Staph infection	Skin or bloodstream infection
Streptococcus pneumoniae	Pneumococcal pneumonia	Pneumonia or bloodstream infection
Candida albicans	Thrush	Vaginal yeast infection, oral yeast infection, or
	Vaginal yeast infection	infection of the esophagus
Coccidioides immitis	Coccidioidomycosis	Pneumonia or widespread infection
	Fungal pneumonia	
	Disseminated fungal infection	
Cryptococcus neoformans	Cryptococcal meningitis	Meningitis
	Cryptococcosis	
	Fungal meningitis	
Cryptosporidium species	Cryptosporidiosis	Diarrhea (intestinal infection)
	Parasitic diarrhea	
Cytomegalovirus (CMV)	CMV retinitis	Eye infection (retinitis), diarrhea (intestinal
		infection), or infection of the esophagus
Herpes simplex virus	Herpes infection	Mouth and skin ulcers, genital ulcers, or infection of
		the esophagus
Histoplasma capsulatum	Histoplasmosis	Pneumonia or widespread infection
	Fungal pneumonia	
	Disseminated fungal infection	
Isospora belli	Isospsoriasis; parasitic diarrhea	Diarrhea (intestinal infection)
JC virus	Progressive multifocal leukoencephalopathy (PML)	Infection of the brain (encephalitis)
Mycobacterium avium complex (MAC)	MAC infection	Widespread infection
Pneumocystis carinii	Tuberculosis	Pneumonia
Toxoplasma gondii	Toxoplasmosis	Infection of the brain (encephalitis)
Treponema pallidum	Syphilis	Genital ulcers or widespread infection
Varicella zoster	Chickenpox; shingles	Rash

Appendices

Index

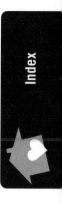

About the Editor

Peter S. Houts is professor of behavioral science and medicine at Pennsylvania State University College of Medicine in Hershey. He is currently director of Family Caregiver Education Program for Central Pennsylvania, funded by the Commonwealth's Department of Health. Dr. Houts is an authority on how illness and medical treatment affects patients and their families. The author of numerous articles on the economic and psychological burden of disease, he has lectured throughout North America and western Europe on the topic of family caregiving for seriously ill patients. The publication of the Home Care Guide series is the culmination of his lifelong commitment to patient education and empowerment. His original work, *American College of Physicians Home Care Guide for Cancer,* provides guidance, information, and realistic solutions that enable patients, their families, and medical staff to solve many health care problems at home. The *Home Care Guide for HIV and AIDS* further refines and elaborates upon this concept.